Health Policy and Practice in Ireland

Health Policy and Practice in Ireland

edited by
Desmond McCluskey

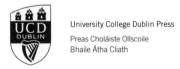

University College Dublin Press
Preas Choláiste Ollscoile
Bhaile Átha Cliath

First published 2006
by University College Dublin Press
Newman House
86 St Stephen's Green
Dublin 2
Ireland
www.ucdpress.ie

ISBN 1-904558-50-X

Cataloguing in Publication data
available from the British Library

Typeset in Ireland in
Adobe Garamond and Trade Gothic
by Elaine Burberry, Bantry, Co. Cork
Text design by Lyn Davies
Printed in England on acid-free
paper by Antony Rowe Ltd

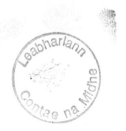

Contents

Health Boards

Important note
The administration of the health services was taken
over by the Health Service Executive in January 2005
and the term 'health board' is no longer in use.

Contributors to this volume

ANNE COLGAN is an independent consultant working with public sector bodies, and voluntary and community organisations. The main focus of her work is on policy analysis and development, including the disability services, education and health. She previously worked as Advisor to the Commission on the Status of People with Disabilities.

JOHN CURRY is a senior officer with the Health Service Executive and lectures on social policy at the Institute of Public Administration and the National University of Ireland, Maynooth. He is author of *Irish Social Services*, now in its fourth edition. He is former chairman of the Commission on Social Welfare (1983–6) and of the Review Group on the Treatment of Households in the Social Welfare Code (1989–91).

GERARD M. FEALY is a Senior Lecturer in Nursing at the School of Nursing and Midwifery, University College Dublin, and is currently Assistant Head of School. He has published numerous papers in the Irish and international academic press. His current research interests include curriculum policy and practice, and the history of nursing.

DONALD W. LIGHT is Professor of Comparative Health Care Systems and Director of the Division of Social and Behavioral Medicine at the University of Medicine and Dentistry of New Jersey, School of Osteopathic Medicine. He has written widely on the practices and ethics of risk-rated health insurance.

DESMOND MCCLUSKEY lectures in the School of Sociology, University College Dublin, and is a member of the Social Science Research Centre, University College Dublin. His principal publications are in the field of medical sociology and the sociology of education.

PETER MURRAY is a Lecturer in Sociology at the National University of Ireland, Maynooth and is Research Associate of the National Institute for Regional and Spatial analysis. He has contributed to major publications on the sociology of health and health economics. Outside the health field, his principal research interests are in the areas of political sociology and the sociology of work.

MARGARET O'KEEFFE is a Lecturer in Sociology in the Department of Humanities at Athlone Institute of Technology. In addition to the research presented here, her interests include the sociology of the mass media.

TONY O'SULLIVAN is a general practitioner in Dublin. He was a founder member of the Irish Patients' Association in 1995, and of Patient Focus in 1997. He has represented the views of health service clients through papers and policy documents and at meetings with the Medical Council and Government ministers.

AOIFE RICKARD is a PhD student in the School of Sociology at University College Dublin. Her Master's degree was on the subject of breastfeeding, and she is now working on a doctoral thesis on sociological aspects of the menopause. She is Assistant Editor of *Figurations*, the research newsletter of the Norbert Elias Foundation.

WILLIAM SHANNON is Professor of General Practice, Royal College of Surgeons in Ireland. He was a founder member of the Irish College of General Practitioners in 1984, and has been one of the main contributors to the development of the teaching of general practice.

ANNE STAKELUM is Senior Qualitative Research Officer with the Department of Public Health in the North Eastern Health Board and is currently on a career break. She has many years of experience as a nurse and midwife.

MÁIRÍDE WOODS is an advocacy executive in Comhairle and is involved in developing an accredited advocacy course with Sligo Institute of Technology and the Equality Authority. She has worked in teaching and research and has undertaken projects in the disability, refugee and education areas.

DERMOT WALSH was Inspector of Mental Hospitals, Department of Health and Children, until 2004. He is currently Principal Investigator, Mental Health Division, in the Health Research Board. He has written widely in the area of mental health.

Abbreviations

ADHD	Attention Deficit Disorder
A&E	Accident & Emergency
BUPA	British Union Provident Association
CME	Continuing Medical Education
CPD	Continuing Professional Development
ERHA	Eastern Regional Health Authority
ESRI	Economic and Social Research Institute
EWTD	European Working Time Directive
FÁS	Foras Aíseanna Saothar
GHDP	General Hospital Development Plan
GMS	General Medical Service
GP	General Practitioners
HBM	Health Belief Model
HIPE	Hospital In-Patient Enquiry
HLC	Health Locus of Control
HMO	Health Maintenance Organisation
HMSO	Her Majesty's Stationery Office
HRB	Health Research Board
HSE	Health Service Executive
ICD	International Classification of Diseases
ICGP	Irish College of General Practitioners
IPA	Institute of Public Administration
ITUC	Irish Trade Union Congress
MHLC	Multidimensional Health Locus of Control
MICGP	Member of the Irish College of General Practitioners
MRCGP	Member of the Royal College of General Practitioners
NAMHI	National Association of People with Intellectual Disability (formerly Mental Handicap) in Ireland
NCCA	National Council for Curriculum and Assessment
NCHD	Non-Consultant Hospital Doctors
NDA	National Disability Authority
NEPS	National Educational Psychological Services
NESC	National Economic and Social Council
NESF	National Economic and Social Forum
NHS	National Health Service (UK)
NRB	National Rehabilitation Board
PAF	Proficiency Assessment Form
PALS	Patient Advocacy and Liaison Service

PHAI   Public Health Alliance of Ireland
PHN   Public Health Nurse
PwDI   People with Disabilities Ireland
RCGP   Royal College of General Practitioners
SVP   Society of St Vincent de Paul
UN   United Nations
VHI   Voluntary Health Insurance
WHO   World Health Organisation

Acknowledgements

I am delighted to take this opportunity to express my sincere gratitude to all of the contributors to this publication; the level of scholarship they brought to the task is evidenced throughout the various chapters and is very much appreciated.

I am greatly indebted to Máire Ní Chearbhaill who acted as consulting editor and who so willingly gave of her time and professional expertise. Special mention, too, must be made of the work of Susan Slattery who was more than helpful in the typing of the manuscript and with advice on its organisation. I can only match her patience and industry with my thanks. I would also like to record my sincere thanks to Niamh Frawley and Mary de Paor who helped me with the typing in the latter stages of the work.

Finally, I would like to register my wholehearted appreciation of the work of Barbara Mennell, Executive Editor of UCD Press, who at all stages of the enterprise was so helpful and encouraging and made my task so much easier.

DESMOND McCLUSKEY
November 2005

Acknowledgements

Foreword

This new edited book by McCluskey brings together a collection of essays which provide a significant sociological contribution to the field of health and health care in Ireland. It adds to a growing body of work in an area which was, until fairly recently, neglected in Ireland. The text is important because of the growing recognition of the need for a more inclusive social model of health and illness. The book carefully outlines the evolution of health policy and the structure of the health care system and provides an important overview of health services. It includes discussion of major political and sociological issues of our time, such as hospital rationalisation, the doctor–patient relationship, health insurance, inequalities in health and health care, power relationships in the organisation and delivery of care, and the treatment and management of people with physical and with mental disability. All of these are hotly debated issues which have clear relevance for health care professionals and policy makers.

The text also points up major educational and training developments which have shaped and which are currently shaping health care in Ireland, such as the changing roles of health care professionals and changing expectations. In addition, it considers health behaviour (such as breastfeeding) and integrates the works of key social theorists into debates which are concerned about such things as local cultural practice, local codes of behaviour and information needs. It concludes with a discussion of lay health beliefs and lay health practices. The book will be a valuable addition to students, scholars and practitioners interested in health, health care and health policy.

DR RONNIE MOORE
*School of Sociology & School of Public Health Medicine
and Population Science, University College Dublin*

Introduction

Desmond McCluskey

Introduction

The most significant factor affecting health policy and practice in recent decades has been the gradual shift of attention away from an exclusively biomedical approach to the understanding of problems of health and illness to a more inclusive social model. In the biomedical model, which predominated in the past, illness is reduced to a discrete biological abnormality inside the body and as Nettleton observes: 'The body is isolated from the person, the social and material causes of disease are neglected and the subjective interpretations and meanings of health and illness are deemed irrelevant' (Nettleton, 1995: 3). The social model, while acknowledging the biological bases of disease, draws attention to the social, economic and environmental causes of health and illness, and health is defined not merely as the absence of disease but as a state of all-round well-being, physical, psychological and social. Further, as McCluskey (1997) notes, a *whole-person* perspective is viewed as central to health care practice, and as a corollary, the patient is to be regarded as an active participant in the therapeutic process, rather than as a passive recipient of medical treatment.

This emphasis on the more inclusive social model is reflected in the policy documents of the Department of Health and Children (formerly the Department of Health). In its publication, *Health: The Wider Dimensions* (Department of Health, 1986) it is stated: 'health is a multi-faceted problem and is linked, to a greater or lesser degree, to all aspects of life'. More recently, the Minister for Health and Children in 2001 launched a National Health Strategy, *Quality and Fairness: A Health System For You* (Department of Health and Children, 2001), to guide activity and planning in the health system for the years 2002–11. In the introduction to the Strategy the social determinants of health are enunciated and their importance in the shaping of health policy is clearly indicated: 'To develop an effective health system, the determinants of health, that is, the social, economic, environmental and cultural factors which influence health, must be taken into account' (2001: 15).

The move in emphasis from a biomedical model of health to a more inclusive social model has had major implications for the education of health care professionals. The study of what are often referred to as the social and behavioural sciences has now become part of the undergraduate curriculum for medical students, and sociology and psychology are core subjects in nursing education. Hence, one of the principal reasons for the preparation of the present publication was to meet the needs of students in the health sciences who are required to study sociology as part of their professional training.

However, the book was designed with other readerships in mind as well. Undergraduate and postgraduate students in sociology who are taking courses in the sociology of health and illness also represent a major target audience. These students will already have a foundation in sociological concepts and theory. It is hoped that the various chapters will advance their interest in health issues and encourage them to pursue these in greater depth. Thirdly, the content of the various chapters is seen as providing a wealth of material for students pursuing postgraduate programmes, not only in medicine and nursing but also in disciplines such as public health, health promotion, social work, health administration and health policy studies.

Finally, the publication should be of interest to scholars outside Ireland who wish to learn about or increase their knowledge of the Irish health care system and the policies and practices on which it is built. The disciplines represented in the various chapters are sociology, social policy, nursing and medicine. The major themes are:

1   Evolution and structure of the Irish Health System
2   Inequalities in health and health care
3   Power imbalances in the organisation and delivery of health services
4   Professional–patient interaction
5   The education and training of health care professionals
6   The health beliefs and health practices of lay people

The book is divided into six sections. Part 1 views health and health care in Ireland from a macro perspective. It focuses on the organisation and development of the health services, on health insurance and on inequalities in health and health care.

In chapter 1, Curry begins with a brief account of the evolution of the Irish Health System from its roots in the nineteenth century. He goes on to review existing services, focusing on the primary care and acute hospital sectors, and in the process highlighting the public/private mix. The contentious issue of hospital rationalisation is traced over several decades, including the context and implications of the recent Hanly Report (Department of Health and Children, 2003b). Curry examines in some detail the background to the administrative changes that occurred as a result of the Health Act 1970 and the proposals for reform of the current structures as outlined in the Prospectus Report (Department of Health and Children, 2003c).

In chapter 2, Walsh traces the changes in the management of mental illness in Ireland from the practice of specialised institutionalism in the nineteenth century to the present policy of community care. Since the introduction of the Mental Treatment Act in 1945, with its emphasis on treatment and care, considerable advances have been made in the psychiatric services and especially so in recent years. Voluntary admission has become a recognised category, new effective drug therapies have been introduced, inpatient numbers have fallen dramatically, the setting up of community-based mental health centres is now widespread, and the shifting of the inpatient base from large psychiatric hospitals to general hospitals is well under way. Finally, Walsh draws attention to the importance of the enactment of legislation in 2001 to safeguard the civil rights of mentally ill persons.

In his analysis of the evolution of Irish health policy, Murray, in chapter 3, presents an overview of the patterns of resource endowment and resource deployment that have characterised the construction of the Irish Health System. The construction of this system was completed by 1970 and within a decade a substantial body of critiques of its performance, which focused on questions of cost, imbalance and inequity, was accumulating. Murray summarises the main lines of this criticism and examines the manner in which state policy has responded to it by bringing forward initiatives to reform the system.

In chapter 4, Light focuses on the issue of health insurance and more specifically on health insurance in Ireland. He contends that it is nearly impossible to construct equitable markets in health insurance that reward efficiencies in services but avoid discrimination against the sick and those at risk. He records how the Voluntary Health Insurance (VHI) scheme, established by the Irish government in 1957 to offer hospital-based insurance to those not eligible for free care, has evolved into a supplementary policy that brings to its members quicker access to hospital care and upgrade of hospital services. According to Light, this evolvement reflects a certain cultural ambiguity, namely, state legitimated two-tier health care, yet carefully protected from the exploitations of risk-rated private care. Light traces developments in the controversy surrounding attempts by the British Union Provident Association (BUPA) to introduce risk-rated health insurance policies and how a counter campaign resulted in the Irish government affirming its commitment to community-based health insurance, thus avoiding the hazards of discrimination.

In chapter 5, McCluskey addresses the issue of health inequalities, focusing specifically on the relationship between health and socio-economic status. He relates that research findings in modern industrial societies, including Ireland, indicate clearly that people from manual working-class backgrounds have higher mortality rates and experience more illness than those from non-manual backgrounds. In discussing the marked inequalities in health between different socio-economic groups, McCluskey notes that the nature of this link has been the subject of much controversy. Though it is agreed that the parts played by lifestyle and material factors are interrelated, he points out that the general consensus among social scientists is that differences in the material circumstances of socio-economic groups are the key determinants of class inequalities in health. Indeed, it is argued that an emphasis on the effects of lifestyles tends to draw attention away from the direct effects on health of the general living conditions of the poor.

Part 2 directs attention to one of most significant developments in health care in Ireland in recent years. It centres on the move in nursing practice away from 'old nursing', which attended to the physical needs of the patient arising out of a medical diagnosis and its associated treatment, to the 'new nursing' perspective which comprehends the patient's psychosocial as well as physical needs.

In chapter 6, Fealy traces the emergence of modern nursing as a secular-professional social practice in the late nineteenth century and reviews nursing's quest for professional regulation in the early twentieth century. The chapter also traces the development of the new clinical roles that nurses established in the last decades of the twentieth century, examining the educational developments that were needed for the expanded nursing roles, and explores the emergence of the graduate nurse at the start of the twenty-first century. Fealy provides a critical analysis of the social factors that underlay the changes in nursing, including the ideologies and the practical imperatives that drove change both from within and outside the nursing profession.

In chapter 7, Stakelum reports on a qualitative study of third-year students in 1994, prior to the end of the apprenticeship model of nurse training, where the role of the student nurse alternated between that of student and of employee. The study is seen as important in that it captures the experience of students socialised within one model of training that can later be used to evaluate the experiences of students within the newer model, where the emphasis is on education rather than on service provision. The study reveals that the experiences of students socialised within the apprenticeship model were characterised by conflict between the respective demands imposed on them by the educational and services segments of training, a situation the students felt powerless to change. The general impression to emerge from the study is that the current model of awarding full student status to student nurses is a move in the right direction.

O'Keeffe's paper, in chapter 8, analyses mothers' views of the Child Health Services and helps throw light on the extent to which the role of the public health nurse (PHN) working in the community is informed by the 'new nursing' perspective. It draws on the findings of a study (McCluskey et al., 1995) of the perceptions of mothers of the services available to them and their infant children. Overall, the mothers were highly appreciative of the work of the PHN. A clear majority stressed the importance of the mother being introduced to the PHN *before* the birth of her baby. This would provide an opportunity for first-time mothers to understand the supportive role of the PHN and allay the fear, articulated by many, that the PHN's main concern was assessing a parent's ability to care for her infant.

Many mothers felt more attention should be given to the mother's own health, in particular her psychological well-being. It emerged, too, that many felt they could be better informed about vaccination and, more specifically, about possible side effects. There was, moreover, resentment at what was perceived as an over-emphasis on breastfeeding, especially in hospital, with very little attention to the difficulties involved. O'Keeffe concludes that the study indicated a rise in a consumerist orientation among mothers.

Part 3 focuses on the doctor–patient relationship. Since no empirical sociological studies on this topic relating to Ireland were available, the editor invited two medical practitioners to contribute their views on the subject. The first contribution is by William Shannon, Professor of General Practice at the Royal College of Surgeons in Ireland and the second by Tony O'Sullivan, a general practitioner and founder member of Patient Focus, a national voluntary patient advocacy group.

In chapter 9, Shannon welcomes the growing acceptance by family doctors of a biopsychosocial model of health, which requires that doctors attend to the biological, psychological and social dimensions of health and illness. For Shannon this change in orientation from the traditional biomedical model means that the doctor–patient relationship will be informed by a patient-centred approach where the patient will take precedence over the disease. He focuses especially on the clinical interview, stressing the importance of attending to the patient's perspective. Shannon rejects the paternalistic model of the doctor–patient relationship in which the doctor is dominant. For him the ideal relationship is one of mutuality, where the doctor encourages and facilitates the patient to participate in decision making.

Like Shannon, O'Sullivan, in chapter 10, is critical of the paternalism which he regards, in many instances, as still characteristic of the doctor–patient relationship. Focusing largely on the negative experiences of patients in hospital care, he identifies four areas from which problems arise. First, patients need to be informed of their rights as soon as they become involved in health care. Second, patients often perceive doctors, especially senior hospital staff, as arrogant – which O'Sullivan sees, in many cases, to be due to doctors' poor communication skills. Third, few Irish health institutions have an adequate protocol for handling the anxieties of patients, their families and health personnel regarding issues of medical neglect and malpractice. Finally, O'Sullivan points to the fact that many specialist services are available only in a few large urban centres, and some only in Dublin, which leads to incalculable difficulties for patients.

Part 4 considers health care in Ireland from the perspectives of two consumer groups. It examines the quality of services available to those with intellectual and physical disabilities and their carers. Woods and Colgan justify the discussion of disability issues in a publication on health policy and practice on the basis that people with disabilities are a significant group of users of the health services and that the Department of Health and Children is the major source of both policy and funding for disability services.

In chapter 11, Woods draws attention to the many advantages accruing to people with learning disabilities resulting from the move from institutional to community care. At the same time, she is highly critical of the level of state support; chronic scarcity, she asserts, still characterises community care in Ireland. Woods acknowledges the major part played by voluntary organisations in the provision of services, including their role in effecting significant changes in the education, training and employment fields. She goes on to identify the very many issues that remain to be resolved and the appropriate actions required. Chief among these are the development and funding of high-quality residential places for adults and the enactment of guardianship legislation in the imme- diate future for those with limited capacity to take decisions for themselves.

Colgan, in chapter 12, in her analysis of the issue of physical disability, suggests that government policy of investing the responsibility for services for people with disabilities with the Department of Health has laid the ground- work for a heavily medicalised approach to such services. As a result, other relevant government departments have not had formalised responsibility for meeting the access, housing, transport or employment needs of people with disabilities. In tracing the state/voluntary sector relationship, Colgan highlights the difficulties confronting voluntary organisations for and of people with physical disabilities. Since they tend to be smaller than organisations in the intellectual disability field, and are more fragmented, there is a real fear that in new organisational and funding arrangements the value and worth of these smaller groups will be overlooked. Colgan observes that, while in the past the focus was on service provision, now the pressure is for a rights- based policy aimed at the building of equality, full participation, independence and inclusion.

Part 5 focuses on lay health beliefs and practices. It discusses Irish attitudes to breast-feeding and analyses the health and illness behaviour of a sample of Irish people.

In chapter 13, Rickard addresses the topic of breastfeeding in the Republic of Ireland, where, she observes, Irish rates compare unfavourably with many other countries. In her analysis, she draws on the work of Norbert Elias, *The*

Civilising Process (1994). From the time of the Renaissance, changes occurred in the social standards governing natural biological functions and many, including breastfeeding, were moved behind the scenes of social life. However, in recent decades rates of breastfeeding have begun to rise, which Rickard suggests reflects a general relaxation of codes of behaviour, especially regarding sexual matters, and in addition a wish by young women to return to nature. However, Rickard argues, owing to the influence of the Catholic Church, the so-called 'permissive society' came late to Ireland and hence feelings of unease in relation to the body, and consequently attitudes to breastfeeding, are not likely to disappear overnight.

In chapter 14, McCluskey reports on a study of the health beliefs and practices of a sample of lay people in Ireland (McCluskey, 1989). In general, the health behaviour of the sample members reflected their perceptions of the main factors associated with good health: eating healthy food, taking sufficient physical exercise and not smoking. However, preventive practices in terms of visits to doctors and dentists for check-ups were infrequent for most people. As emerged from other studies, health and illness behaviour were found to be related to socio-demographic factors. Women, generally, were more likely than men to take actions in the interest of their health. So, too, middle-class sample members were more likely than manual working-class respondents to report that they behaved in ways regarded as conducive to good health. The latter appeared to be higher utilisers of medical services when ill, but, as McCluskey notes, evidence from other studies suggests that lower-income people use fewer services relative to their needs.

Several important analyses of health care in Ireland have appeared in recent years. Among the most notable have been Barrington's study (1987) of the conflicts associated with the development of the Irish health services from 1900 to 1970; Hensey's review (1988) of the evolution of health care in Ireland, and Wren's critique (2003) of the Irish Health System. However, a comprehensive sociological analysis of health and health care in Ireland still remains to be undertaken. A beginning was made with the publication in 1997 of *The Sociology of Health and Illness in Ireland* (Cleary and Treacy, 1997). The present work, which complements that of Cleary and Treacy, is intended as a major contribution to this project. While the views expressed here are not necessarily those of the editor, they provide a wide range of perspectives on issues relating to health care in Ireland.

Part 1

Health and health care in Ireland:
A macro perspective

Chapter 1

Overview of the health services

John Curry

In recent years there has been an unprecedented analysis of the Irish Health System and if the recommendations emanating from this are implemented, the Irish system will undergo considerable change in the coming decade. The Health Strategy, *Quality and Fairness: A Health System for You* (Department of Health and Children, 2001a) was the cornerstone of the analysis, providing a comprehensive blueprint for developments for reform of the health services over a ten-year period, setting out core principles, national goals and objectives for implementation through over 100 actions. Arising from the Health Strategy, three key reports, Prospectus, Brennan and Hanly,[1] published in 2003, set the basis for the most fundamental changes in the system for over thirty years. The principal administrative change was the abolition of regional health boards and their replacement on 1 January 2005 by a single agency, the Health Service Executive. The purpose of this chapter is to give an overview of the Irish health services. It includes an introductory historical section, key features of, and issues associated with, some of the main services; financing; the system of eligibility for services; and an outline of the administrative system.

In an overview chapter such as this it is not possible to include an analysis of the range of existing public health services. Instead, there is a selective focus on the primary care sector (with particular emphasis on general medical practitioner services) and on the acute hospital sector. These sectors cater for the majority of health consumers and also account for a large proportion of the total health budget. Only some of the key issues related to these two sectors are considered.

---

[1] The full titles of these reports are *Audit and Functions in the Health System* (usually referred to as the Prospectus report after the main authors, Prospectus management consultants) (Watson Wyatt Worldwide, 2003); *Commission on Financial Management and Control Systems in the Health Service* (usually referred to as the Brennan Report after the chairperson of the Commission, Professor Niamh Brennan), and *Report of the National Task Force on Medical Staffing* (usually referred to as the Hanly report after the chairman, David Hanly) (Department of Health and Children, 2003b).

Evolution of health services

A useful starting point for considering the evolution of health services in Ireland is the nineteenth century, where it is possible to distinguish between four main strands: hospital services, mental hospital services, dispensary services and prevention services.[2]

The hospital system had emerged over a period with some voluntary hospitals established in the eighteenth century, initially by philanthropic individuals and later by religious orders. These hospitals were usually located in the larger urban areas, mostly Dublin. Some have provided a service well into the twentieth century and beyond. In addition to the voluntary hospitals, a network of public infirmaries and fever hospitals were developed. By the 1830s there were approximately 20 county infirmaries and 70 fever hospitals. A further component in the hospital system was the workhouse whose medical role gained in importance as the numbers in the workhouses declined towards the latter part of the nineteenth century.

Treatment of mental illness was confined to lunatic asylums. A few large asylums were established in the nineteenth century. Among these was the Richmond Institution at Grangegorman in Dublin, established in 1815, which continued to function well into the twentieth century as St Brendan's Hospital (see Robins, 1986; Reynolds, 1992). In addition to these large institutions, district asylums were established in almost all counties.

The Poor Law was introduced in Ireland in 1838 as a nationwide system of alleviating destitution. The central feature of the Poor Law was the workhouse but some other services were developed outside the workhouse, the most notable being the dispensary system. Under this system, introduced under the Poor Relief Act 1851, a network of dispensary districts was established throughout the country, in each of which a doctor was employed to provide a free service to the poor of the area. This dispensary system continued well into the twentieth century and was the forerunner of the present choice-of-doctor scheme for medical cardholders.

Health preventive services were limited throughout most of the nineteenth century, with the result that outbreaks of infectious diseases had serious consequences, especially for the population of urban areas (see Robins, 1995). By the latter part of the nineteenth century the link between public and personal hygiene and the transmission of disease became firmly established by scientists. This, together with the work of public health reformers, resulted in the Public Health Act 1878 and the introduction of measures to ensure proper sanitation, clean water supplies and food hygiene controls. Subsequent advances were such that, 'by about 1900 large scale epidemic disease had become history' (Robins, 1995: 241).

---

2   This section draws substantially on Hensey (1988).

Apart from the evolutionary development of the above and related services to meet changed circumstances and advances in medicine, a number of broad trends were discernible in the health services throughout the twentieth century. Firstly, there was a gradual shift away from the community as a focus of health care to the health needs of the individual. Some of the early measures in the nineteenth century were designed not so much to promote individual health as to prevent community-wide catastrophes through the spread of infectious diseases. Similarly, in mental illness the emphasis was on protecting society rather than on rehabilitating the individual. Secondly, the state became more and more directly involved in the planning and provision of health care. This did not occur without controversy and opposition from the Catholic Church and the medical profession. The classic instance of this was the Mother and Child Scheme that Dr Noel Browne, Minister for Health (1948–51), proposed to introduce. The Catholic hierarchy opposed the scheme (which would have provided free health service for women before, during and after childbirth and for children up to 16 years) on the grounds that it represented undue state intervention. The medical profession opposed the scheme because it did not want a comprehensive state health service, preferring instead a mix of public and private.[3]

Thirdly, there was a move away from local administration to a more centralised model. The myriad of local administrative units in the nineteenth and early twentieth centuries was gradually rationalised. The number of such units was reduced from 90 in the 1920s to eight following the Health Act 1970. At central level, Health emerged as a separate government department in 1947 out of the former Department of Health and Local Government, which had been established in 1924 (it was renamed the Department of Health and Children in 1997). Fourthly, the administrative changes at local and regional level reflected a change in funding from local taxation (rates based on property valuation) to central funding. At the beginning of the twentieth century, the health services were largely funded from local taxation, a system whose shortcomings became increasingly apparent. A gradual shift towards central funding occurred over several decades so that by the late 1970s, local taxation no longer contributed to financing and the services were funded almost entirely through the exchequer from general taxation and a special health levy. The progressive involvement by government throughout the twentieth century has been summarised by Barrington:

In 1900, governmental responsibility for the health of the population was limited to controlling outbreaks of the most serious epidemic diseases and ensuring access

---

3 There are various accounts of the controversy surrounding the Mother and Child Scheme. These include relevant sections in Barrington (1987); Browne (1986); Deeny (1989); Whyte (1980), Horgan (2000).

by the poor to general practitioner services and Poor Law infirmaries. By 1970, government had accepted responsibility for providing a high standard of medical care for all sections of the population at no or at a heavily subsidised cost to the recipient (Barrington, 1987: 279).

Primary care sector

It has been noted that 'primary care is the first point of contact that people have with health and personal social services' (Department of Health and Children, 2001b: 7). For the most part this means first contact with a general medical practitioner who provides services to both private and public patients, the latter being medical cardholders and their dependants.

The general practitioner service for medical cardholders under the community care programme is part of the General Medical Service (GMS), which accounts for about one third (31.8 per cent) of expenditure on the total community care programme or just under 10 per cent of the entire non-capital health expenditure. This service is vital to the primary health care needs of almost one third of the population.

General Medical Service

As already noted, a free general practitioner service for poor persons was provided from 1851 in local dispensary districts. This system continued until 1972. The White Paper, *The Health Services and their Further Development* (Department of Health, 1966a), had referred to the advantages of the dispensary system but indicated that the segregation of the population into fee-paying patients (who attended the doctor's surgery) and public patients (who attended the dispensary) outweighed any of its merits. Consequently, the 1970 Health Act provided for the introduction of a choice-of-doctor scheme under which eligible persons would not be discriminated against in regard to place of treatment. The choice-of-doctor scheme comes under the General Medical Service (GMS), which also subsumes the service provided by pharmacists to those eligible. The scheme, introduced in 1972, gave eligible patients – medical cardholders and their dependants – the choice-of-doctor to the greatest extent practicable and ended the discrimination and stigma attached to the dispensary system.

In 2003, there were 2,181 doctors and 1,292 pharmacists participating in the scheme. Most of the doctors care for both private and eligible patients, although the ratio between both categories of patients may vary considerably between parts of the country since there is a wide divergence in the distribution of medical cardholders. Under the dispensary system, most of the doctors supplied drugs, medicines and appliances to eligible patients. Under the GMS, retail pharmaceutical chemists are the primary channels of supply of drugs prescribed for eligible persons. Prescriptions are dispensed without charge to the patient and the pharmacist recoups the cost of the drugs and, in addition, is paid a dispensing fee.

Since its inception in 1972, expenditure on the GMS has been a matter of some concern, especially the cost of providing drugs and medicines that have accounted for about two thirds of the total expenditure on the GMS annually. The *Report of the Working Party on Prescribing and Dispensing in the General Medical Service* (Working Party, 1974) noted that a number of doctors over-prescribed to a significant extent – prescribing too many items, prescribing excessive quantities and constantly prescribing the more expensive drugs without regard to their cost. A further working party report (Working Party, 1984) examined methods by which the GMS might be made more cost-effective, with a special emphasis on the way in which doctors were paid.

Under a new system of payment introduced in 1989, participating doctors receive a capitation payment in respect of each panel patient, weighted by reference to demographic characteristics (age and sex), and geographic factors (distance of the doctor's principal place of practice from the patient's home). Prior to this participating doctors were paid a fee-per-consultation.

In 2003, according to the *Report of the General Medical Service (Payments) Board* for the year ended 31 December 2003, the cost per eligible person was €247 (doctor cost), and €562 (pharmacy cost), giving an average total GMS cost of €809 for every person with medical card eligibility (as compared with €679 in 2002). With reference to the GMS costs per eligible person, the Deloitte & Touche report, *Value for Money Audit of the Irish Health Services* (Deloitte & Touche, 2001) indicated that the GMS, 'represents real value for money' and 'the cost per person per year is relatively low' (2001: 25).

The Health Strategy (Department of Health and Children, 2001a) proposed the introduction of an interdisciplinary, team-based approach to primary care provision. A more detailed account was published in *Primary Care: A New Direction* (Department of Health and Children, 2001b), which acknowledged that the primary care infrastructure is poorly developed and that there is little teamwork and limited availability of many professional groups. It indicated that members of the primary care team would include GPs, nurses/midwives, health care assistants, home helps, physiotherapists, occupational therapists, social workers and administrative personnel. While a 'one-stop shop' is the ultimate goal, it is acknowledged that because of buildings and infrastructural implications, team members may not be housed together initially. Development along the lines proposed would make an important difference to the quality of primary care services for patients.

Acute hospital sector

This acute hospital sector covers the treatment of patients in medical, surgical and maternity hospitals, including outpatient clinics associated with these hospitals. These services are provided either directly by the Health Service Executive (HSE) in hospitals under their control or by contract with voluntary and private hospitals. There are three categories of hospitals: public, voluntary public and private. Public hospitals are owned, funded and managed by the HSE on behalf of the government and treat some private but mostly public patients. Voluntary public hospitals are those established and owned by religious orders or other foundations; they are funded by the HSE and treat both public and private patients. Private hospitals do not receive any government funding and cater exclusively for private patients. Given the manner in which the hospital system evolved it is not surprising that rationalisation would be an issue.

The first report of the Hospitals Commission (Department of Local Government and Public Health, 1936), covering the period 1933 to 1936, favoured the grouping of hospitals in suitable geographic centres 'irrespective of county boundaries'. It submitted a scheme for the development of 12 main regional centres, county hospitals in areas remote from regional centres, and a network of district hospitals in the provincial towns. The Commission was critical of the situation in Dublin where there were too many small hospitals and it recommended the development of two general hospitals in south Dublin and two in north Dublin. These proposals were not pursued, partly because the government had already embarked upon the development of county hospitals, and also because the large number and unique role of voluntary hospitals in Dublin made change more difficult (see Barrington, 1987: 120–1; Daly, 1999).

In 1968 the report of a consultative council on hospital services was published, usually referred to as the Fitzgerald Report (Consultative Council on the General Hospital Service, 1968). It indicated that the existing hospital system was defective in staffing, equipment, quality of service and teaching standards. It suggested that the system could only be improved by a radical reorganisation involving, among other things, a considerable reduction in the number of centres providing acute treatment and a planned and co-ordinated hospital organisation embracing both the public and voluntary hospitals. It recommended that the hospital system be reorganised into three regions based on the medical teaching centres in Dublin, Cork and Galway. Each region would have a regional hospital of 600 to 1,000 beds, offering a full range of services, supported by a number of general hospitals of about 300 beds throughout the region. General practitioners catering for non-acute cases needing care would staff the existing district hospitals. The existing county hospitals were to be community health centres providing inpatient services as suggested for district hospitals but backed by increased diagnostic facilities and a more comprehensive consultant outpatient organisation. Reaction to the report in the centres not selected for development was predictably hostile (see Barrington, 1987: 266–9).

Not surprisingly, in view of widespread opposition, there was no official commitment to implement the Fitzgerald Report. In 1973 Brendan Corish, TD, Minister for Health, initiated a process of widespread consultation, involving the medical profession, health boards, and Comhairle na nOspidéal, (established under the Health Act 1970 as an advisory body on hospitals). Guidelines drawn up by Comhairle modified the earlier recommendations of the Fitzgerald Report and proposed that the general aim should be to organise acute hospital services with specified minimum staffing so that the population served would be within a radius of 30 miles of the hospital centre.

Following a process of consultation with all of the interested parties, the *General Hospital Development Plan* (GHDP), sometimes referred to as the Corish Plan, was published in 1976. It differed fundamentally from the Fitzgerald Report in the number of acute care hospitals to be established. The GHDP envisaged the development of general hospitals in 23 locations (about twice as many as envisaged in the Fitzgerald Report). The major differences between the GHDP and the Fitzgerald Report were distance of population from a general hospital (30 miles versus 60 miles) and, related to that, the number of centres in which general hospitals should be located (23 versus 12). By comparison with the Fitzgerald Report, the GHDP plan could be viewed as a balance between professional medical opinion and broader political considerations. However, *The Irish Times* put it somewhat differently:

> Indeed, it is not so much a national plan of any substance as an interim political statement on the state of play at local level. (*The Irish Times*, 21 October 1975)

Both the Fitzgerald Report and the GHDP gave rise to concern and opposition in those communities whose hospitals would lose some of their services. The word 'downgrade' became synonymous with either loss or a diminution of local hospital services. The status of the local hospital has remained a live local political issue ever since and has been a successful platform for some 'hospital candidates' in local and national elections.

It was in the context of cutbacks in public expenditure on the health services that a rationalisation of hospitals occurred in the late 1980s. During this period a number of the public voluntary hospitals and the smaller public district hospitals were closed, often amid considerable controversy. The most notable example was that of Barrington's Hospital in Limerick, a public voluntary hospital that had been established under charter in 1830. Approximately 6,000 beds were removed from the system in the late 1980s and early 1990s with a reduction from 17,665 in 1980 to 11,832 in 2000 (Department of Health and

Children, 2002). Not all of this occurred as a result of a coherent national plan. The closures of some hospitals was brought about by the Department of Health, either reducing budgets to health boards, thus leaving them with no option but to close the smaller hospitals, or by simply informing a number of voluntary public hospitals (funded directly by the Department) that they would have to close. Rationalisation of hospital services in Dublin was a protracted affair that took several years to complete, partly because in some cases it involved the amalgamation of existing hospitals with different traditions and ethos. This was particularly true of Tallaght Hospital, opened in 1998 in the southwest suburbs, as an amalgam of three former city hospitals, the Adelaide, Meath and National Children's hospitals.

Hanly Report

The most recent proposals with implications for the configuration of hospitals are contained in the Report of the National Task Force on Medical Staffing (2003), usually referred to as the Hanly Report. The Task Force was established to consider the implications of the European Working Time Directive (EWTD) under which the working week for non-consultant hospital doctors (NCHDs) must be introduced in stages: 58 hours by August 2004, 56 hours by August 2006 and, finally, 48 hours by August 2009. The Hanly Report indicated that there were over 3,900 NCHDs working an average of over 75 hours. There were 1,731 consultants, to whom patients had limited access.

To meet requirements of EWTD, different options were considered by the Task Force, for example, it would be necessary to employ an additional 2,500 NCHDs to ensure all worked within time limits set out in EWTD. The preferred option was to employ a much larger number of consultants working in teams, with revised working patterns and a significantly reduced number of NCHDs. The Hanly Report indicated that 'hospitals without sufficient volume of patients and activity cannot sustain large numbers of consultants' and that 'best results in treatment are achieved when patients are treated by staff working as part of a multi-disciplinary specialist team' (National Task Force on Medical Staffing, 2003: 15). In short, the Hanly Report recommended a consultant-provided as opposed to the existing consultant-led hospital service.

The Task Force examined two regions (East Coast Area Health Board and Mid-Western Health Board) and proposed a reconfiguration of hospital services. In the Mid-West region the report concluded that Limerick regional hospital should function as the major hospital for the region while Ennis, Nenagh and St John's (Limerick) should function as local hospitals. The local hospitals would not have 24-hour accident and emergency service.

While the recommendations of the Hanly Report stemmed from logical positions adopted by the Task Force regarding the best possible patient care, these views were not shared by the communities affected. Apart from positive reaction from government and certain other sections, it was like the Fitzgerald Report and GHDP all over again as the highly emotive term 'downgrade' re-entered the vocabulary of national and local politics. Within a relatively short time, reaction to the proposals at local level became clear. Public protest meetings in Ennis and Nenagh attracted estimated crowds of 20,000 and 10,000 in November 2003 (*The Irish Times*, 17 November, 1 December 2003). Opposition to and criticism of the Hanly proposals have also been voiced by some hospital consultants.

Against a background of growing local opposition and, in particular, the formation of a national alliance in March 2004, the Health Services Action Group, representing local hospital action groups from across the country, it is likely that the implementation of certain aspects of the Hanly Report proposals will be modified.

Eligibility for health services

Since June 1991, the population falls into two categories for eligibility for health services. In Category I is the lowest income group – medical cardholders and their dependants – accounting for 30 per cent of the population, with entitlement to all health services free of charge. The remaining 70 per cent are in Category II and are entitled to a more limited range of services.

The main difference between the two groups is that while the medical card population (Category I) is entitled to a free general practitioner service and hospital service (in public wards of public and voluntary public hospitals), the rest of the population (Category II) is liable for general practitioner fees but is entitled to a 'free' hospital service (subject to a maximum annual charge of €550) on the same basis as the medical card population.

Prior to 1991 the system was highly complex, with the population divided into three categories. This situation had evolved over a considerable period. From 1851 the low-income group had eligibility for health services under the dispensary system of the Poor Law and in 1953 the middle-income group obtained limited eligibility for services, leaving the higher group without any entitlement. In 1979 further reforms were introduced to simplify the system of eligibility but the three-tiered system remained until 1991. An attempt was made in 1974 to rationalise the system into two categories (as at present), but this was stymied because of the opposition of hospital consultants.

It is important to note that there is no statutory basis for determining eligibility based on the two categories above. Persons with full eligibility for health services (medical cardholders and their dependants) are defined in the Health Act 1970 as 'adult persons unable without undue hardship to arrange general practitioner, medical and surgical services for themselves and their dependants'. Prior to the establishment of regional health boards in 1970, the criteria used in assessing means were not uniform in all health authority areas. Entitlement to a medical card is based on assessment of means, and income limits for determining eligibility are revised annually to take account of inflation.

With improvements resulting from the introduction of the choice-of-doctor scheme in 1972, the number of persons covered by medical cards increased up to the late 1980s (table 1.1). In 2003 there were 1.16 million persons, representing almost 30 per cent of the total population. A number of factors account for the increase throughout the 1970s and early 1980s. These include the abolition of the dispensary system to which a certain stigma was attached; the introduction of uniform guidelines to determine eligibility and the increase in the social welfare population mainly due to the increase in unemployment. The proportion of the population covered by medical cards has declined steadily since the late 1980s, from 37.4 per cent in 1988 to 29.6 per cent in 2002 (the latter being only slightly higher than the proportion thirty years earlier when the choice of doctor scheme was introduced). This decline is partly attributable to the general improvement in the economy, the consequent real increase in average per capita incomes and the drop in unemployment.

In July 2001 eligibility for medical cards was extended to all persons aged 70 or over, irrespective of income. The Health Strategy (Department of Health and Children, 2001a) indicated that eligibility would be extended to increase the number of persons on low incomes and priority would be given to families with children and particularly children with a disability. In line with this, a commitment was made by government in 2002 to increase the medical card population by a further 200,000 persons. No progress was made until 2004,

Table 1.1 **Number of persons and percentage of population covered by medical cards, selected years, 1972–2003**

	No. of persons covered by medical cards	Percentage of total population
1972	864,106	29.0
1976	1,193,909	37.0
1980	1,199,599	35.6
1986	1,326,048	37.4
1988	1,324,849	37.4
1990	1,221,284	34.9
1996	1,252,385	34.6
2003	1,158,143	29.6

Source: General Medical Service (Payments) Board, *Annual Reports*.

when the government announced proposals to increase the number of medical cardholders by 230,000 from the beginning of 2005. However, 30,000 of these will be entitled to a medical card in the traditional sense (covering GP visits and prescribed drugs), while the remainder are to receive a card that entitles them to GP visits only. This will result in a two-tiered medical card system.

Health insurance

The Voluntary Health Insurance Board (VHI) was established as a non profit-making body under the Voluntary Health Insurance Act 1957 to enable those in the higher income group, who did not have eligibility to health services at the time, to insure themselves against the cost of medical care. The virtual monopoly enjoyed by the VHI in health insurance ended when, at the instigation of the EU, competition was provided for under the Health Insurance Act 1994. This allowed BUPA (British Union of Provident Assurance) to enter the Irish market in 1997 and Vivas in 2004. Health insurance companies operate a community rating system, that is, all age categories are charged the same premium even though the risk of ill health obviously varies depending on age (see Light, chapter 4).

The White Paper *Private Health Insurance* (Department of Health and Children, 1999), set out a programme for change which included the transformation of the VHI into a commercial semi-state agency and the retention of a revised system of community-based rating. It also proposed the establishment of a Health Insurance Authority to regulate the market (Department of Health and Children, 1999). The Health Insurance Authority was established on a statutory basis in 2001.

It is estimated that membership of health insurance schemes accounts for approximately 47 per cent of the population, with the VHI having by far the largest share of the market (Amárach Consulting, 2003). It is clear therefore that a large number of persons in Category II, with an entitlement to subsidised hospital care in public hospitals, have invested in supplementary cover to enable them to have private or semi-private accommodation and private treatment by consultants in hospitals. The reasons for this include the faster access to hospital and avoidance of waiting lists (Department of Health and Children, 1999). This highlights the public/private mix in the Irish Health System. The introduction of the choice-of-doctor scheme in 1972 ended the differences in access between public and private patients to general practitioners, but the difference in access to hospital services has grown rather than diminished over the same period. Waiting lists are associated with public rather than private patients (see McCluskey, chapter 5).

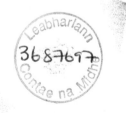

Financing of health services

The major source of income for expenditure on current health services is the exchequer (table 1.2); up to 1977, however, local taxation was an important and significant source of income. During the nineteenth century, local rates constituted the primary source of income for health services and only towards the end of the century were state grants provided. By 1947, state grants accounted for 16 per cent of the total cost of the services. Developments in the health services post-Second World War necessitated increased expenditure. Under the Health Services (Financial Provisions) Act 1947, the state undertook to meet for each health authority the increase in the cost of its services until the cost of the services provided by the authority was being shared equally with the exchequer. The White Paper of 1966 indicated that local rates were not a form of taxation suitable for collecting revenue on the scale required for proposed developments in the health services and recommended instead that the cost of further extensions of the services should not be met by the local rates. By 1970, the exchequer's contribution amounted to 56 per cent of total costs. In 1973 the government decided to remove health charges from local rates over a four-year period and by 1977 the transfer had been completed.

Another source of revenue, the health contribution, was introduced under the Health Contributions Act 1971 at the request of the Department of Finance which was concerned at the falling contribution from local rates. Since 1991 the contribution (currently two per cent) is levied on a person's total income. It is important to note that payment of the contribution does not give entitlement to any health service. A further source of income since 1973 is derived from receipts under EU regulations. These receipts are mainly in respect of health services provided for people for whom Britain is liable under EU regulations, for example recipients of British pensions and dependants of persons employed in Britain.

An important source of revenue for hospitals for several decades was the Hospitals Trust Fund. A number of voluntary hospitals joined forces to run a sweepstakes from horse racing following the First World War. The venture proved successful and under the Public Hospitals Act 1933 available surpluses of ensuing sweepstakes were to be payable to the Hospitals Trust Fund, appointed by the Minister for Health and Local Government to administer the funds. The income from the Fund was used mainly for capital expenditure on all hospitals. The role of the Hospitals Trust Fund in financing hospital development and services had declined considerably in importance when the sweepstake was abolished in the early 1980s. Despite a controversial history, during which the proportion of funds raised for hospitals from the sale of tickets dwindled while the administration and associated costs rose, the 'Sweepstake' made a significant contribution to the development of hospitals (Barrington, 1987: 284; J. McAnthony, *Irish Independent*, 6 December 2003).

Commission on Health Funding

The Commission on Health Funding was established in 1987 against a background of expenditure cutbacks in public services and particularly in the health services, and growing disquiet among health service unions and the public at large with the consequences of these cutbacks. The Commission's report, published in 1989, examined not only the financing of the health services but also the administration and delivery of services. It concluded that the level of public health funding could not be determined by reference to a fixed proportion of Gross Domestic Product or by reference to international comparison. In the Commission's view the level could be decided only in the context of the available resources and the priorities attached by Irish society to different social objectives.

The Commission referred to three main methods of funding health services: general taxation, social insurance, and private insurance. It pointed out that no country relies exclusively on any one of these approaches. The majority of the Commission favoured public funding as the main funding method in preference to private funding on the basis that the state as central funder was favourably placed to plan and organise the delivery of a unified, integrated service for all categories of patient (Commission on Health Funding, 1989: 81).

Having opted for a public funding model, the choice was then between general taxation and a compulsory health insurance/earmarked tax system (linking the services provided with their cost). A majority favoured general taxation on the grounds that compulsory health insurance was effectively another tax, offering no real advantages over general taxation. The Commission recommended that the existing health contribution should be abolished. Apart from this, the Commission effectively favoured the status quo in relation to funding of the health services.

Almost 90 per cent of funds for health services are derived from the general taxation through the exchequer with the health contribution and hospital outpatient charges accounting for just over 10 per cent (table 1.2).

Table 1.2 **Sources of finance for statutory non-capital health services, 2001**

	€m	%
Exchequer	5,830	86.5
Health contributions and miscellaneous	723	10.7
Receipts under EU regulations	186	2.8
Total	6,739	100.0

Source: Department of Health and Children, 2003a.

Administration

The evolution of the administrative structure for health care in Ireland up to
recent decades has been outlined in admirable detail by Hensey (1988). Here
the main focus is on developments since the establishment of health boards in
1970, with an emphasis on current reforms. As already noted, the trend during
the twentieth century was towards a reduction in the number of agencies
with responsibility for the administration of health services. This rationalisation
process was progressed over several decades and culminated in the replacement
of 27 local health authorities (based on counties) by eight regional health boards.
The reasons for the regionalisation of health functions in 1970 were outlined in
the White Paper 1966 (*The Health Services and Their Further Development*,
Department of Health, 1966a). One of the principal reasons was that the
county was too small a unit for the provision of a range of specialist services.

Under the Health Act 1970, the health services were to be administered by
eight health boards, each covering a number of counties. The population of the
regions varied with, for example, the Eastern Health Board (counties Dublin,
Kildare and Wicklow) having a population approximately six times that of
either the Midland (counties Laois, Longford, Offaly and Westmeath) or
North Western (counties Donegal, Leitrim and Sligo) Health Board areas in
1971. The density of population and the location of existing facilities, especially
hospitals, however, explain some of these differences.

The membership of each health board represented a combination of three
main interests:

- Elected representatives drawn from county councils and borough councils
- Professional representatives of the medical, nursing, dental and pharma-
  ceutical interests and
- Nominees of the Minister for Health (three on each board).

The change from a county to a regional system of administration in 1970 was
not achieved without some concessions, and Erskine Childers, TD, Minister
for Health, had bowed to political pressure by conceding just over half the
membership of health boards to local elected representatives (Barrington, 1987:
274). In the majority of cases, an elected local representative has been
chairperson of each health board (a non-executive position filled on an annual
basis) since their establishment.

With the exception of the eastern region, the health board structures
established in 1970 were to remain unchanged for over thirty years. In 2000, the
Eastern Regional Health Authority replaced the Eastern Health Board and a
number of consequential changes occurred to the structures in the eastern region
as well as membership of the Authority. In 1986 the Department of Health had

summarily raised the question as to whether eight separate administrations were necessary given the size and population of the country but did not follow through on this (Department of Health, 1986).

The role of health boards was analysed in some depth in the *Report of the Commission on Health Funding* (1989). While the Commission was established to review funding of health services, it concluded that the solution to the problem facing the health services lay not so much with funding as with the way services were planned, organised and delivered. The Commission identified a number of weaknesses in existing structures, for example a confusion of political and executive functions, and a lack of balance between national and local decision making.

One of the main problems cited by the Commission was that many voluntary agencies providing health services (including voluntary hospitals and some of the larger voluntary organisations providing services for people with disabilities) were not funded by health boards and therefore did not report to them: instead they were funded directly by the Department of Health. The Department of Health and the Minister for Health were consequently involved in the management of services rather than concentrating exclusively on developing and monitoring policy. In order to overcome these and other weaknesses, the Commission recommended that

- the Minister for Health and the Department of Health should formulate health policy and should not be involved in the management of individual services.
- The management of the health services should be transferred to a new agency, the Health Services Executive Authority. The Authority would be responsible for the management and delivery of health and personal social services in the context of health policies set by the Minister for Health.
- Existing health boards should be abolished and be replaced by Area General Managers, with responsibility for the delivery of services within defined geographical areas.

Government did not accept these radical proposals for the replacement of health boards. However, the validity of the diagnosis was accepted in part and led to reform of structures in the eastern region. In 1991, Dr Rory O'Hanlon, TD, Minister for Health, referred to failings in the health service structure as identified by the Commission on Health Funding and the Dublin Hospital Initiative Group. These included the lack of co-ordination between hospital and community-based services, the resultant over-involvement of the Department of Health in day-to-day management issues, and the lost opportunities for achieving efficiencies through greater co-operation between agencies. He indicated that the fragmentation of services and the lack of co-ordination were particularly acute in the Dublin area because of the multiplicity of autonomous agencies involved in the provision of health care and he proposed the establishment of a new structure. The most significant structural reform of the health services since the Health Act, 1970 occurred with the establishment of the Eastern Regional Health Authority by legislation in 2000. As part of the restructuring, the former Eastern Health Board (covering the counties of Dublin, Kildare and Wicklow with a total population of 1.3 million in 1996) was replaced by three Area Health Boards – the East Coast Area Health Board, the Northern Area Health Board and the South Western Area Health Board covering the same geographic area, with the Eastern Regional Health Authority having overall responsibility for health and personal social services provided by both statutory and voluntary agencies in the region. The health board structures in other parts of the country were not altered.

Some other deficiencies in the health system as identified by the Commission on Health Funding were also addressed. The Health (Amendment) (No. 3) Act 1996, often referred to as the accountability legislation, strengthened and improved the arrangements governing financial accountability and expenditure procedures in health boards, and began the process of removing the Department of Health from detailed involvement in operational matters. The process of funding voluntary public hospitals and the main voluntary organisations for people with intellectual disabilities through health boards, rather than directly by the Department of Health and Children, commenced in 1998.

The Health Strategy (Department of Health and Children, 2001a) proposed a review of structures that was subsequently undertaken by Prospectus and Watson Wyatt Worldwide in consultation with the Department of Health and Children. The report, *Audit of Structures in the Health System*, published in 2003 and usually referred to as the Prospectus Report, recommended radical changes to existing structures. These recommendations were resonant of those in the report of the Commission on Health Funding but went further. In its analysis of the existing system, the Prospectus Report identified a number of weaknesses. Among these were the following:

• The health system was characterised by fragmentation of structures and functions, with too many agencies (58 in total), often operating independently of each other.
• The Department of Health and Children still had an involvement in the day-to-day operation of the system.
• There was poor integration of services which 'often make for a difficult journey for an individual patient or consumer across the system's component parts'.
• The traditional health board model had evolved over the years in an unstructured manner and had resulted in insufficient co-ordination and standards.

• Tensions between local representative decision making and the delivery of national and regional strategic objectives hindered decision making.

The Prospectus Report argued that because of these and related weaknesses in the system, there was a need to develop a consolidated structure to deliver on a range of priorities.

In order to create this structure the Report recommended the following:

• The abolition of health boards and the establishment of a Health Service Executive to manage the health services as a single national entity.
• The establishment of three core areas within the Health Service Executive: a National Hospitals Office, a Primary, Community and Continuing Care Directorate and a National Shared Services Centre.
• The establishment of four regional health offices within the Health Service Executive to deliver regional and local services.
• The establishment of a Health Information and Quality Authority to promote quality of care throughout the system.
• The abolition or merging of a number of other health agencies.

In 2002, the Minister for Finance established a Commission to examine the various financial management systems and control procedures operated by the Department of Health and Children and health boards. This arose from growing concern regarding efficiency and productivity in the health service, where there had been an allocation of substantially increased financial and staff resources over the previous few years. The key recommendation of the Commission on Financial Management and Control Systems in the Health Service (Brennan Report) was the establishment of an executive to manage the health services on a unified national basis. Both the Prospectus and Brennan reports, with different terms of reference, had therefore concurred on the central solution for reform of the health services.

These proposals for reform of health structures were endorsed by government and were outlined in *The Health Service Reform Programme* (Department of Health and Children, 2003c). In November 2003 an interim board of the Health Service Executive (HSE) was appointed by Micheál Martin, TD, then Minister for Health and Children. He indicated that the HSE would assume responsibility for health services from January 2005. Opposition to the abolition of health boards, especially by elected representatives who constituted the majority on health boards, was muted. There was a general acceptance in many circles of the need for structural reform. The Health Act 2004 provided for the establishment of the Health Service Executive which replaced the former health boards and some other agencies and assumed responsibility for health services from 1 January 2005.

Conclusion

Various political, economic and social factors have helped to shape the present health services. A distinguishing characteristic that has emerged is the mix of public and private provision of health care and the consequent existence of a two-tier system. Much of this stems from the traditional role and influence of the voluntary hospital sector.

The structure of the health care system now seems sets for fundamental change. The process of rationalisation of the number of administrative units throughout the twentieth century has been taken a step further with the establishment of one health agency, the Health Service Executive, for the entire country. In time, this and associated changes should ensure the consistent implementation of policies throughout the country and make a significant difference to the quality of service provided.

Chapter 2

Mental illness in Ireland and its management

Dermot Walsh

Whereas in earlier times insanity and the insane might be matters of curiosity with esoteric speculation as to their origins, by the mid-eighteenth century insanity, together with mental deficiency, or idiocy and imbecility as they were more commonly called in those days, had become a matter of considerable social concern, in Europe at least. The reason for this was, in all probability, demographic in origin. The eighteenth century in Europe was a time of considerable population expansion. This in turn was the consequence of the Agricultural Revolution or the improvement and greater sophistication of agriculture. The introduction of root and grain crops ensured an abundance of nutritious, efficiently produced foodstuffs on a scale hitherto unavailable. As a consequence, human resistance to those infectious diseases which periodically devastated European populations and ensured, through high mortality rates in early life, that the majority of people born did not live to adulthood and which preyed upon the undernourished, the weaklings and the sickly, so often the product of their nutrition, now took a much lower toll of better nourished, and therefore more disease-resistant peoples. Thus diseases like plague, smallpox, cholera, dysentery and, notably, tuberculosis, although still the main causes of death in Europe, were less ravaging and better contained than previously. In such changing circumstances, infant and early life mortality decreased and many more persons lived to adulthood or even old age. Before these changes it is reasonable to assume that the mentally ill and the mentally handicapped, by reason of their increased susceptibility to the major fevers and, because of less enthusiastic attempts to ensure their survival by comparison with the mentally normal, ensured an excess mortality for these groups of people. Therefore, it may be reasoned that they did not survive in sufficient numbers to adulthood to constitute a social problem. In the altered circumstances of the eighteenth century all this changed.

As the century progressed and the agricultural revolution was followed by the Industrial Revolution with the establishment of large towns and cities and the population shift from countryside to urban settings, it may be assumed that, in spatial terms alone, these disadvantaged groups became even more of a burden to their families and the community as a whole. Large factories sprang up with knowledge of the uses to which iron, steel and coal might be put. Factories sprang up on the Ruhr and in the industrial north of England. Over the nineteenth century, families, including young children, went to work in conditions that were depicted by Dickens in England and Zola in France in graphic and frightening terms. In such circumstances no one was available to look after the mentally ill and the mentally handicapped.

Private sector response

Despite growth in what later came to be described as 'the lunatic poor', it was perhaps not surprisingly the private sector which first responded to lunacy among its numbers. By the early eighteenth century most of the great families of Europe had already been established, some tracing their origins back to the late Middle Ages. Over this time, of course, they had accumulated great wealth and property and this was passed on in lineal descent in most countries through primogeniture: to prevent the breaking up of great estates and to ensure their provision in their entirety these passed on to the eldest son of the family, a process which was not to survive the French Revolution in that country. Any threat to the process by which property was preserved through descent in perpetuity within the same family had obviously to be dealt with appropriately and harshly. The two great threats to wealth and continuity were illegitimacy and lunacy and both were legislated against. Both could obviously lead to the dissipation of what had been built up over centuries, wealth passing out of the family through illegitimacy and dissipated through the mental incapacity to manage. On the other hand, it became necessary to establish laws to ensure that neither the one nor the other could inherit property. It was established thus by law that the illegitimate could not inherit. Legislation to this effect enacted at that time has persisted virtually to the present day in most European countries including our own. Similarly, laws to enable the mentally ill to be committed to 'private madhouses', where by reason of such commission they would be deprived of the right to manage their own affairs, were instigated at this time. And for the mentally handicapped or 'imbecilic' or 'idiotic', the possibility of their being registered as 'wards of court' was established, so that their affairs would be managed by others.

So it was that by the mid-eighteenth century private mad houses were established throughout Europe to cater for those whose relatives had the means to cover the expense involved. Such madhouses were established in Ireland as well as elsewhere and even those such as St Patrick's in Dublin, which were set up for charitable purposes, were in large measure only capable of catering for those with means because of the cost involved. The largest and the most enduring of these private or charitable institutions in Ireland was established by the Dean of St Patrick's Cathedral, Jonathan Swift, whose Gulliverian fantasies, parodies and moral instruction are well known to us. The relevant case, the establishment of St Patrick's, he wrote with more wit than scientific accuracy:

> He gave the little wealth he had
> To build a house for fools and mad
> To show by one satiric touch
> No nation needed it so much
> (Jonathan Swift, 'Verses on the Death of Dr Swift' in Bequest of Jonathan Swift)

The traditions and practices which draw a line between the wealthy mad and the lunatic poor endure to this day.

Public sector response

Towards the second half of the eighteenth century the lunatic became recognised as a public order nuisance because of vagrancy, begging and petty criminality. Much of this derived from their being excluded from family and orderly society and so they had to resort to other means of self-support. The constabulary and the magistrates dealt with them through the criminal law exercised through the minor courts. And so they found themselves in bridewells and jails to whose occupancy they made a not insubstantial contribution. By the early nineteenth century the fact that they had increased in numbers, that they were seen as contributory to social disorder, that they were recognised as constituting a distinct subclass within society and that much of their petty criminality was driven by forces outside the common moral code, all contributed to the dawning of the requirement for a distinct and autonomous response to the problem they posed.

Even though Dublin had a house of industry providing for lunatics at the turn of the nineteenth century and Swift's hospital was still admitting the pauper poor, although these were eventually to be entirely replaced by paying patients, little else was available for the lunatic poor. Accordingly, in 1804 a Committee of the House of Commons, although looking at the distressed poor generally, recommended that separate provision in four provincial asylums be made for the lunatic poor. A bill was prepared as a first step to putting this recommendation into effect but it was eventually lost in terms of commanding parliamentary attention and finally disappeared altogether. In Dublin it was resolved in or around 1810 that a separate lunatic asylum should be established, and in 1815 the Richmond Asylum, named after the Lord Lieutenant of the day, the Earl of Richmond, opened its doors for business. In 1817 a Select Committee of the House of Commons was given the task of advising the government on making further provision for the lunatic poor in Ireland. Noting that – besides the provision made by the Richmond Asylum – other accommodation was available on a formal or informal basis elsewhere in the country for idiots and the insane, such as the Cork Asylum, the Select Committee reported that existing accommodation was clearly inadequate, and that some of the accommodation available in houses of industry was a social disgrace. It proposed that lunatic asylums be established on a district basis and that as a beginning four or five should be set up with a capacity of over a hundred patients each. This recommendation was given effect by an Act passed in 1817 providing for the establishment of the asylums as recommended. However, providing enabling legislation for the establishment and management of asylums and financing their erection were two different things so it was many more years before the national system of district lunatic asylums came into being. However, asylums began to appear on a district basis, beginning with Armagh in 1824 and followed in succeeding years by Limerick, Belfast and Derry in the 1820s and by Ballinasloe, Carlow, Clonmel, Maryborough (Portlaoise) and Waterford in the 1830s.

The first wave of asylum building was to variations around a common plan devised by the celebrated architect Richard Johnson for the Board of Works, the institution responsible for public building in the country. The basic principle of design underlying these first asylums was that of the philosopher and social reformer, Jeremy Bentham (1748–1832) and revolved, literally, around the Panopticon. This consisted of a central column, rather like a lighthouse, with observation from the top storey and which served as the spine of the building out from which radiated the individual wings of the asylum. Probably the best example of this was at Limerick District Asylum. In others a frontispiece of classical design fronted the radiating wings and usually contained the administrative offices, as at Carlow and Maryborough. In all of these first-wave asylum buildings the design was classical, the accommodation on two floors and in individual cells.

Inspectorate of mental hospitals

From 1770 the welfare of lunatics in houses of industry and in jails had been entrusted to the inspector of prisons. However, in the 1840s a medical man much interested in the welfare of lunatics, Dr Francis White, successfully lobbied for a separate inspectorate of mental hospitals. He himself had been associated with the Richmond Asylum for over ten years. His petitioning was successful and in 1846 he took up office as the first Inspector of Lunacy in Ireland. He was assigned an administrative headquarters in Dublin Castle and given the necessary clerical infrastructure to carry out his task which, as well as providing detailed statistics on lunatics in Ireland, necessitated the compilation and presentation of a report to the Lord Lieutenant on the state of lunacy in Ireland at the end of each year.

It became apparent that as soon as the District Lunatic Asylums were open and operating they filled to capacity. And this, despite the fact that ancillary provision for lunatics and idiots was provided through the policy of a national system of workhouses or poorhouses for the relief of the indigent poor, expeditiously accomplished between the years 1838 and 1841. By the time White had taken office there were probably as many lunatics and idiots in workhouses as in district lunatic asylums. Indeed, White himself had instigated in 1844 a series of surveys on lunatics and idiots at large, usually carried out by the local constabulary in each district. According to White, the first of these had estimated over six thousand lunatics and idiots at large, the majority of them being vagrant. It was necessary therefore, according to Dr White and his assistant, the Assistant Inspector of Lunacy, Dr Nugent, to expand considerably the asylum system to accommodate them. As lunacy report after lunacy report to the Lord Lieutenant urged, more accommodation became necessary and so a second wave of asylum building began in the 1850s, and at the same time the existing asylums were everywhere extended. These asylums, again commissioned by the Board of Works, were to be on three storeys, in a broad Gothic revival style and providing accommodation in dormitories rather than in single cells and they were designed by a variety of different but distinguished Irish architects of the time. In 1852 the Cork or Eglington asylum replaced the existing building and that year also saw the opening of new asylums at Killarney and Kilkenny, to be followed by Omagh in 1853, and Mullingar and Sligo in 1855.

Despite their fresh extensions and new building the inspectors judged the asylums to be still overcrowded and so a third and final wave of building began which extended from the late 1850s (Sligo) to Portrane in Dublin in 1895 and Antrim in 1899. These latter asylums were built in a variety of different styles from the Elizabethan revival to the Florentine palazzo – all of them with some degree of architectural distinction.

Retrospectively it was clear that the Victorians had, largely at the instigation and through the energy of the inspectors, responded to the lunatic problem by a policy of specialised institutionalisation. At the outset, lunatics were accommodated in houses of industry, in jails and were at large in considerable numbers. By the end of the nineteenth century virtually all 20,000 of them, constituting 0.5 per cent of the Irish population, were in the district lunatic asylums provided for them. A few lingered on in former workhouses until well into the twentieth century but these were the exceptions and probably over-represented the mentally handicapped and the elderly. Notwithstanding this, approximately one fifth of those in district lunatic asylums were mentally handicapped rather than mentally ill, a situation which was not to change throughout the next half century.

Life in the asylum was ordered, regular and pretty unchanging from day to day. The asylums were self-contained entities surrounded by high walls containing within their precincts all that was necessary for daily life. Thus, there were bake-houses, butcheries, vegetable gardens, sewing rooms where clothing for inmates was created, cobblers' shops and so on. The whole community was held together by the medical superintendent, senior nursing personnel, further medical personnel and then the great body of attendants. Day-to-day running of the institution, in its visible sense, was the responsibility of an ample trade and labouring staff. Virtually all of these functionaries were accommodated in housing provided either within the grounds of the asylum or close by. Thus, although the wages were not of any great consequence, the attendant benefits such as housing, fuel and provisions made up for the meagreness of the cash reward. At a time when unemployment was rife in Ireland and when emigration was the rule for many members of families, employment in the asylum system was highly prized and descended within families, with intermarriage between male and female staffs being the rule rather than the exception. Of course, throughout, the genders were separated within the asylum, each having its male and female house and each gender being cared for by its own so that it was a serious offence for a male, for example, to enter the female house. The economic importance of the asylum system can be gauged from the fact that the population of the town of Ballinasloe in 1951 was 5,596 persons of whom 2,078 were patients in the asylum, a situation which was not that different from that of a hundred years previously.

Twentieth-century developments

The asylums continued on their peaceful way, with those in what was to become Northern Ireland passing to that jurisdiction, or rather remaining in the old one, with the foundation of the Irish Free State in 1922. Nothing very much happened in the asylum system during the first half of the twentieth century with the exception of the last purpose-built asylum, St Brigid's, Ardee, being provided for County Louth. In the 1930s no major building project was undertaken. Neither in physical status, nor in matters of legislation or innovative treatments did any great change occur. In fact, as far as the first half-century (1900–45) was concerned, the asylum system actually stood still.

New mental health legislation became law in 1945 with the introduction of the Mental Treatment Act of that year. This replaced the Lunacy Law (Ireland, 1903) and the changing emphasis in mental health services towards 'treatment' was enshrined in the title of the new Act. This was despite the fact that very few effective treatments were available prior to 1945; in this respect at least, legislation was looking forward rather than backwards. While much of the 1945

Act was concerned with technical matters of administration and employment it did break new ground in relation to administration procedures and detention. A new form of detention was introduced which was time-limited to six months in the first instance although this was extendable to a total period of two years. In addition, voluntary admission became a recognised category for the first time in a formal sense (it was possible to be a voluntary boarder in a private institution prior to the introduction of the 1945 Act). When the Act became operative in 1947 it took some time for the voluntary admission status to become widely used, and in the early years the percentage of patients admitted voluntarily was still in the minority before climbing to constitute approximately 90 per cent of all admissions, as is the case today.

In the 1950s attempts were made to set up outpatient clinics at general hospitals so that patients suffering from psychiatric disorders could receive treatment other than as inpatients, the exclusive situation until this time. In addition, a small number of clinics placed in general hospitals were also instigated as, for example, at Mercer's Hospital in Dublin, where the psychiatric clinic was operated by the staff of St Brendan's Hospital, Grangegorman. Both the legislative innovation of voluntary admission and the setting-up of outpatient clinics away from the mental hospital base were driven by the requirement, increasingly recognised, of making access to psychiatric care, both in hospital and in the community, more readily available. The extent to which such provision was visionary is exemplified by the fact that by 2000 almost 90 per cent of the 24,282 admissions in psychiatric hospitals and units were on a voluntary basis. In this same year there were no fewer than 230,723 attendances at psychiatric outpatient clinics throughout the country (Daly and Walsh, 2001). About this time, too, the old district mental hospital boards, which were responsible for the running of mental hospitals and represented joint authorities, usually county councils, were disbanded in favour of health authorities, so that, for example, in the Dublin area the psychiatric hospitals were the responsibility of the Dublin Health Authority.

New drugs, new treatments

By the 1950s electro-convulsive therapy became widespread in the treatment of depression and of other illnesses. No doubt it was used more often than was necessary, and inappropriately in some cases, but it nevertheless was of great value to persons suffering from depression and in many cases was dramatically rapid in the relief that it provided for this condition. At the same time the insulin treatment of schizophrenia, later to be abandoned, was in full vogue. In the middle of the decade the so-called major tranquillising drugs were introduced, marking a huge step forward in the treatment of psychiatric disorder.

Finally, towards the end of the 1950s, the introduction of anti-depressant drugs, as an alternative or adjunct to electro-convulsive therapy, further stimulated therapeutic psychiatric activity. All of these treatments, arriving in the 1950s, gave an impetus to therapeutic treatment activity in psychiatric services. Psychiatrists were stimulated by the new horizons that had begun to reveal themselves to them, and whereas by 1958 the number of patients in Irish psychiatric hospitals had reached a record total of 21,000, these numbers began to fall thereafter year-on-year to the present day.

Commission of Inquiry on Mental Illness

In 1966, the *Report of the Commission of Inquiry on Mental Illness* expressed serious concern about the numbers of Irish people in psychiatric hospitals.

> In Ireland, approximately 7.3 psychiatric beds were provided in 1961 per 1,000 of the population; this rate appears to be the highest in the world and compared with 4.5 in Northern Ireland, 4.6 in England and Wales, 4.3 in Scotland, 2.1 in France and 4.3 in USA. At any given time, about one in every seventy of our people above the age of 24 years is in a mental hospital. When it is remembered that every mentally ill person brings stress into the lives of people around him, it will be clear that in Ireland mental illness poses a health problem of the first magnitude (Department of Health, 1966b).

Because numbers in Irish psychiatric hospitals were running at a rate of approximately 0.7 per hundred of population and because, both from the Inspector of Mental Hospital reports, which continued on an annual basis, and from anecdotal evidence, the belief was well-founded that physical conditions in many Irish psychiatric hospitals were poor, and that in international comparison hospitalisation rates were twice those of neighbouring countries, the government of the day decided to set up a full-scale Commission of Enquiry on Mental Illness in 1961. The commission was given the broad brief of examining and reporting on conditions in Irish psychiatric services and of making recommendations for their improvement. This body presented its report to government in 1966. Among its principal findings and recommendations were that the psychiatric services were largely institutional in nature; that child psychiatric services were virtually non-existent; that clinical support staff such as social workers, psychologists and occupational therapists scarcely existed in services; that staff training was neglected and that many professionals lacked the necessary skills for the tasks which they should have been carrying out. The Commission stressed the importance of providing alternatives to hospitalisation such as day hospitals, day centres, the establishment of community-based psychiatric residences and group homes. It saw the future of psychiatric inpatient care as being general hospital-based and saw the decline of the large psychiatric hospital. It recommended that staff be increasingly trained in community-based work, that social workers, psychologists and occupational therapists be recruited to provide true interdisciplinary team care and that psychiatric services be instigated and developed throughout the country.

The Commission would like to have examined the question of whether the high number of hospitalised patients in Irish psychiatric services represented a higher level of mental illness in the Irish community than in other countries but found that the data to enable such an enquiry to take place did not exist. Accordingly, it recommended that the Medico-Social Research Board should develop a mental illness/mental health database for this purpose. With the setting up of the Medico-Social Research Board in 1967 this became a reality.

Mental illness: categorisation and classification

Attempts at the classification of mental illness have been of major concern to psychiatrists and others for years. With the arrival of 'scientific' psychiatry in the nineteenth century, further attempts to identify and separate types of mental illness from each other were regularly undertaken, usually with limited success. It was not until the turn of the century that a statement by a German psychiatrist, Emil Krapelin, led to the fundamental distinction between two major forms of 'madness' not due to evident injury or damage to the brain through infection or other known causes. These were called, respectively, manic-depressive illness, primarily a disorder of mood, and dementia praecox, a disorder of early life in which the fundamental thinking capacity of an individual becomes deranged, with other secondary symptoms and difficulties arising from this. This latter condition was to be renamed schizophrenia by the Swiss psychiatrist, Evoem Bleuler, in 1911. There followed in the next half-century the recognition of illness owing to obvious damage to the brain, whether by infection or by trauma, or by degeneration leading to the condition called Alzheimer's Dementia recognised in 1903 and largely seen in elderly people and characterised by a decline in all mental faculties but particularly in memory and judgement. These so-called 'organic' diseases of brain, among which syphilis was a major causative factor before its virtual elimination by penicillin, were distinguished from the so-called 'functional' illness in which no evidence of infection, damage or degeneration was obvious in the brain and which largely comprised schizophrenia and manic-depressive disorder (or bipolar disorder as it came later to be known). These two groups of illnesses together constituted the psychotic group of illnesses because in them there is serious impairment with the thought and mood functions not seen, or at least not seen to such an extent, in other psychiatric disorders. Other disorders comprised two major groups: the neuroses characterised by conditions of anxiety including phobia and obsessions, on the one hand, and a group whose status has long been debated – that of the personality disorders – in which basic personality traits evident in every human being are exaggerated to a degree sufficient to interfere with successful living in all its aspects.

The specialised health agency of the United Nations, the World Health Organisation (WHO), was established in New York in 1946. The mental health division of WHO was deeply concerned with the matter of diagnosis and classification in psychiatric disorder because of the disarray that existed in this matter at national level. At one point in the 1960s, WHO employed a consultant to review the matter internationally. The disappointing outcome was that there were almost as many different classificatory systems as there were countries in which psychiatry was practised. To overcome this difficulty, WHO devoted a major portion of its mental health budget towards standardisation of diagnosis and classification in psychiatry to enable international communication and comparisons in research work to be undertaken in this field. In its International Classification of Diseases (ICD), WHO devoted an entire section to psychiatric disorders and this has gone from revision to revision, currently being in its tenth revision. As a result of these efforts there is no doubt that the process of diagnosis and classification in psychiatry has greatly improved internationally, enabling meaningful interchanges and communication in epidemiological work to take place in this discipline.

The Medico-Social Research Board, later to become the Health Research Board, adopted the new classificatory systems in psychiatry and each year returns detailed information concerning patients who were admitted to or discharged from psychiatric hospitals in units throughout the country, as well as information on patients in community psychiatric services. This information has been found to be very useful in monitoring trends and in helping planners in setting up and improving mental health services.

Table 2.1 presents the numbers of patients in Irish psychiatric hospitals, both public and private, and in psychiatric units in general hospitals, aged 16 years and over on 31 March 2001 by diagnostic categories arranged in accordance with the classification of the tenth edition of the International Classification of Diseases (Daly and Walsh, 2002).

Table 2.1 **Diagnosis of inpatient population 31 March 2001. Numbers, percentages and rates per 100,000 population aged 16 years and over.**

Diagnosis	Number	%
Organic psychoses	317	7.3
Schizophrenia	1701	39.4
Other psychoses	49	1.1
Depressive disorders	752	17.4
Mania	424	9.8
Neuroses	146	3.4
Personality disorders	125	2.9
Alcohol disorders	241	5.6
Drug dependence	56	1.3
Mental handicap	392	9.1
Unspecified	118	2.7
All diagnoses	4,321	100.0

Source: Daly and Walsh (2002)

The future: moving towards community care

The *Report of the Commission of Enquiry on Mental Illness* (Department of Health, 1966b) was bullish enough to suggest that, if its recommendations were implemented, the number of beds needed for acute psychiatry would fall from 21,000 or thereabouts in 1960 to 8,000 in 15 years' time, that is, from the presentation of its report in 1966 to the year 1981. While the Commission's report was clear and incisive in its examination of the existing situation and in what it proposed should be done about it, it had one major defect: it did not outline nor even indicate what mechanisms should be put in place to ensure the implementation of its recommendations. The consequence was that although improvements occurred in mental health services, these were often patchy and local, rather than comprehensive and general. Thus, the first psychiatric unit based in a general hospital opened in Ardkeen Hospital in Waterford in 1967; the number of outpatient clinics increased; here and there day hospitals were set up; rehabilitation services were put in place and a social worker and a psychologist or occupational therapist or two were employed; yet overall progress was slow and was not as the Commission had envisaged. The consequence was that by 1981, instead of being at 8,000, the number of occupied psychiatric beds had fallen only to 16,000, twice that envisaged by the Commission.

Because the recommendations of the Commission of Enquiry on Mental Illness had been implemented only to a limited degree, an advisory group or working party on psychiatric services was set up towards the end of 1981 with much the same brief as had been the Commission's twenty years earlier. Its report at the end of 1984, *The Psychiatric Services: Planning for the Future* (Department of Health, 1984) essentially endorsed and extended these recommendations. Additionally, it dealt in some detail with the matter of the implementation, suggesting in each service that management teams might be set up to this end, what their constitution might be and how in detail they should apply themselves to their task.

In 1992 the Department of Health issued a Green Paper on mental health which reminded readers that the Programme for Economic and Social Progress set out a number of priorities for psychiatric services:

- The continued development of specialist assessment in rehabilitation units associated with the main acute general hospitals
- Additional places in day centres, workshops and supported hospitals
- The further development of child and adolescent psychiatric services
- The development of community alcoholism programmes
- The further development of alternative approaches to the delivery of psychiatric services.
- The transfer of people with mental handicap inappropriately placed in psychiatric hospitals into the main handicapped services (Department of Health, 1992: 3).

Acknowledging that health boards had plans for the advancement of their psychiatric services, as recommended in *Planning for the Future*, the Green Paper undertook to review progress to date. In addition to outlining once again and reaffirming commitment to the recommendations of the Commission report and *Planning for the Future*, the Green Paper (Department of Health, 1992) identified particular groups for which specialised services might be necessary. These included disturbed patients, patients or persons with psychiatric illness coming before the courts or in prison, the elderly mentally ill and persons with substance abuse problems. It stressed the importance of sectorised psychiatric services, whereby specific sectors of approximately 30,000 of the population within an overall catchment area of psychiatric services were to be the responsibility of multidisciplinary psychiatric teams. This policy of sectorisation would ensure continuity of care and the integration of primary health care services with specialist psychiatric services. The Green Paper devoted over half its length in Part II to a review of mental health legislation, a topic that will be returned to shortly.

Progress in the delivery of mental health care since 1984

The fact that considerable progress has been made towards the objectives of policy in relation to psychiatric services is evidenced by the fall in psychiatric inpatient numbers from 19,801 in 1963 to 4,321 on 31 March 2001 (Daly and Walsh, 2002). The root cause of this decline of inpatients has been the reduction through mortality of the old long-stay patients and their non-replacement by new long-stay patients. This latter influence has been largely the consequence of the extension of community-based alternatives to hospitalisation, particularly long-term hospitalisation. That further reductions are inevitable over the next decade or so is exemplified by the fact that of the existing inpatients almost half are over age 65 and these long-stay persons will be greatly reduced by mortality in the coming years. The setting-up of community-based mental health centres in each sector out of which multidisciplinary teams work, rather than using the inpatient base as a centre of activities as was previously the case, is now widespread throughout the country. The shifting of the inpatient base away from the large psychiatric hospitals is now well under way, and during 2000 general hospital psychiatric units accounted for almost 40 per cent of all admissions. As a result of these developments, two of the largest psychiatric hospitals in the country, in Sligo and Cork, have been sold and major parts of other hospitals have been acquired by other, mainly educational, services while yet others have been the subject of negotiation with local authorities, who saw in the substantial facilities that they offered potential for new uses. At the same time, much hospital land, including hospital farms, had been sold with substantial profit to the health boards, which since 1961 had been providing public psychiatric services. Much of the money derived in this way was ploughed back into improving psychiatric services.

The extension of community-based alternatives to hospitalisation meant that in some services, up to half of the nursing staff were working in community-based rather than inpatient services. In 2000 there were almost a quarter of a million attendances at outpatient services nationally (Daly and Walsh, 2001). There were 2,427 day-centre places providing for over 5,000 persons, with an additional 1,192 day-hospital places providing for over 17,000 patients. Health boards provided, during 2000, a total of 2,934 community residential places (Daly and Walsh, 2001). The patients living in these group homes and hostels were a mixture of rehabilitated and discharged long-term patients and newer patients who had become homeless or, for other reasons, were in need of alternative residential accommodation.

Progress in relation to the provision of child psychiatric services was slow but steady. At the end of 1996 there were upwards of 15 psychiatric teams in place throughout the country. A growing speciality of psychiatric services for the elderly was also evidenced by the existence of four full-time specialist teams being in place at the end of 1996.

Mental health legislation

With over half a century elapsed since the 1945 Mental Treatment Act, it was inevitable that practice in mental health services would outstrip legislation. By the 1990s the outdated nature of the legislation under which services were provided had become very evident. An attempt had been made in 1981 to introduce a new Mental Health Act but although the Bill had become an Act and had gone through all the necessary preliminaries, it was never implemented. This was because when an attempt was made to draft the regulations governing its operation, serious operational difficulties were discovered. That new legislation was imperative was indicated not alone by the outmoded nature, in practical terms, of the 1945 Act in relation to current conditions, but also because numerous international bodies had issued statements setting out principles governing the rights of mentally ill patients which needed to be enshrined in legislation. Details of these and of suggestions as to the content of new mental health legislation were set out in the *Green Paper on Mental Health* (Department of Health, 1992) which was essentially a discussion document inviting submissions on its content. Having taken these into account the Department of Health proceeded to draft the *White Paper on Mental Health* legislation which appeared in 1994. Thereafter, the Bill was passed by both houses of the Oireachtas in July 2001 and was then signed into law by the President.

The Act allowed for the establishment of a Mental Health Commission and this was put into place in early 2002. Among the issues dealt with under the new Act, the civil rights of mentally ill persons are central. In practice, these are to be safeguarded by Mental Health Review tribunals which will examine each individual detention as to its legality. The Act provides for shorter periods of involuntary detention, specifies that informed consent will be an indispensable component of the administration of any treatment and that involuntary detention will be automatically reviewed in all cases periodically, whether the detained person requests it or not.

Conclusion

Psychiatric care in Ireland has undergone radical change since the 1960s when the Commission of Enquiry on Mental Illness reported that psychiatric services were largely institutional in nature, that child psychiatric services were virtually non-existent and that clinical support staff were rarely to be found. Since then there has been a dramatic drop in psychiatric inpatient numbers; the establishment of community-based mental health centres out of which multi-disciplinary teams work is now widespread; there has been a steady increase in the provision of child psychiatric services, and action has been taken to safeguard the civil rights of mentally ill persons. Further, the shifting of the inpatient base away from the large psychiatric hospitals is well advanced; it is envisaged that by the year 2010 every psychiatric service will have an acute unit in a general hospital – already 40 per cent of such units are operational and an additional 20 per cent are built and ready to operate. It is to be hoped that psychiatric care will be a top priority in future government health plans and budgets, that the expansion of services will continue apace, and that further progress will not be inhibited by inadequate funding or lack of political will.

Chapter 3

The evolution of Irish health policy: a sociological analysis

Peter Murray

Health and health care provision have become universal public policy concerns in the twentieth century. But the precise nature of these concerns differs from state to state. The history of how a country's health care service system has come to acquire a specific shape plays an important role in defining the kinds of problems its present-day policymakers find themselves grappling with. Moving from a focus on the universal to a focus on the particular, three key questions are encountered. First, what capacity do the state of available scientific knowledge and the existing level of technological application of this knowledge give human societies to tackle problems in the health field? Second, given the differing levels of development and wealth creation that exist between different societies, what is the size of the resource base from which a particular society sets out to meet its health and other needs? Third, given that even between societies that have similar wealth levels, differently structured and regulated arrangements for utilising resources to tackle health problems have become entrenched over time, and that strengths and weaknesses are likely to be associated with any specific set of arrangements, how should policymakers set about developing the former and eliminating the latter?

This chapter is primarily concerned with policy issues arising within the particular Irish context but it will seek to develop a fuller understanding of that context by drawing upon the insights of scholars who have brought a comparative perspective to bear upon the study of the health care systems universe. It begins by situating the universality of health and health care policy concerns within the wider context of continuous social and technological change set in train by industrialism. It then surveys the availability of resources for health care services in Ireland, and the manner in which those resources came to be deployed as the system of services completed by the 1970 Health Act was put in place. The body of critiques of the performance of this system which accumulated during the 1980s is then discussed. Finally, the extent to which the critiques of the 1980s have prompted responsive initiatives since 1990 is examined. Here the measures taken during the decade to secure an increased return of 'health gain' from the resources expended on health services are surveyed and assessed.

Health care and industrialisation

The growth of professionally staffed health care systems is a global feature of twentieth- century society. An important part of the institutionalisation of scientific and technological advance within industrialised societies is medicine's diagnostic and therapeutic armoury which has increased over time in technical sophistication, effectiveness and cost. Innovations diffuse rapidly across national boundaries. Methods of diffusion include international linkages within professions, marketing of patented new drugs or equipment by business organisations and – particularly in the case of the developing word – development aid programmes (Rogers, 1995). To see how health care system growth fits into the wider picture of technological and social change it may be helpful to consider in outline a key formulation of what Goldthorpe (1992: 411) terms 'the theory of industrialism that has prevailed – or, at all events, has had by far the greatest currency – within western social science over the last three decades'. This is 'the logic of industrialism' of Kerr et al. (1973) which is summarised in figure 3.1.

Figure 3.1 **The logic of industrialism**

Workforce	Increased skills and widening range of skills; increasing occupational and geographical mobility; higher levels of education more closely related to industrial function; structured work force
Scale of society	Urbanisation and decline of agriculture as a way of life; larger role for government
Consensus in society	Increasing ideological consensus in a pluralistic society
Worldwide industrialism	Industrial society spreads out from the centres of advanced technology

Source: Kerr et al. (1973), chart 1.

The chain of the logic of industrialism is made up of the following links. First, Kerr and his associates believe that the operation of industrial technology demands a workforce with a high level and wide range of skills. The range and complexity of the tasks workers are required to perform mean that this workforce must be a 'structured' one within which there are many specialised occupations. Second, to recruit such a workforce, society has to be open and allow great scope for social mobility. It is necessary, in other words, for every position to be filled on merit. This means that talented individuals born into poor families can rise to positions of wealth and power while the slow-witted offspring of rich families are at the same time allowed to descend into subordinate and relatively poorly paid positions. An individual's career comes to depend on what he or she knows, not on whom he or she is connected with. Third, in an industrial society people acquire their skills and demonstrate their merits mainly through the acquisition of educational qualifications. Education systems expand therefore in all industrial societies and they are expected to provide industry with the type of skilled manpower it needs.

Fourth, the use of industrial technology gives rise to economies of scale. This term refers to a situation in which the more units you produce the cheaper the average cost of producing each individual unit becomes. Where economies of scale obtain, production on a large scale enjoys an advantage of efficiency over small-scale production. When industrial technology is utilised by a society, workers become concentrated in a small number of large centres of production. Society becomes highly urbanised and the government has to become increasingly involved in providing economic infrastructure such as roads or airports and social services like housing, health and leisure facilities. Because of this, the role played by the state in society expands. Fifth, industrial technology promotes a common set of values – science and technical knowledge come to enjoy high prestige while change is accepted and is viewed as representing ongoing progress towards a generally better state of affairs – across the societies which utilise it. Sixth, industrialism fans out from the centres of advanced technology to affect all parts of the world, bringing with it a set of common values whose increasingly general acceptance will underpin a lessening of international conflict.

The concerns of the present paper draw attention not to the logic chain as a whole (for an appraisal of which in relation to the Irish case, see Goldthorpe, 1992) but to its fourth link. Here, health care is enumerated as an item of essential industrial society infrastructure in whose provision there is expected to be a strong degree of government involvement. The more advanced a society is along the path to industrialism, the better it would generally be expected to perform in putting a comprehensive health care infrastructure into place for its members. As to the degree of government involvement in this task, one of the key findings of comparative studies of national health care systems is that for all societal wealth/development levels, there is a crucially important variability in the extent to which, and manner in which, this occurs. A country's level of affluence and the degree of government control exerted over its health care system are indeed the two key dimensions of variation around which an influential framework for the comparison of health care systems around the globe has been constructed by Light (1994). This framework, which is reproduced in figure 3.2, highlights two aspects of the role played by government in this field. The first is whether or not it assumes the main responsibility for the provision of funds to the health care system out of the revenues it collects. The second is whether or not it directly (by owning facilities, employing personnel) or indirectly (by laying down conditions to which the activities of privately owned facilities and self-employed personnel must adhere to) exerts a strong degree of control over the care service providers. From universal considerations, this chapter now turns to consider how societal wealth and governmental control characteristics have featured in the particular historical shaping of the Irish Health System.

Figure 3.2 **Health care systems by societal wealth and regime of control**

| | The degree of governmental control | | | |
	Decentralised......................Centralised			
Affluence (GNP/capita)	*Private insurance, private, entrepreneurial services*	*National insurance, private, regulated services*	*National insurance, public, regulated services*	*National insurance state-run system*
Affluent	United States	Germany Canada	Great Britain Norway	Former East Germany Former Soviet Union
Wealthy but developing	—	Libya	Kuwait	—
Modest and developing	Thailand	Brazil	Israel	Cuba
Developing poor	Ghana	India	Tanzania	China

Source: Light (1994).

Development of Irish health care

In her standard work on the development of the Irish health care services, Barrington (1987: 281) concludes that advances in medicine, the widening of democracy and rising living standards are 'necessary conditions' of the changes that occurred between the beginning of the century and 1970. But she also concludes that the specific form the changes took can only be accounted for in relation to 'the particular historical, social and cultural experience of the country' before and during that period. The Poor Law system established by the British government in the 1830s, together with the profusion of voluntary hospitals established under either Protestant or Catholic auspices, were a legacy from history that left a distinct imprint on the modern system of services. With much of this initiative dating from a period when the country had a population twice as large as the twentieth century, the system was from the outset over-loaded with expensive to maintain, but politically difficult to cull, institutional care settings. As well as the infirmaries of its workhouses, the Irish Poor Law system – unlike the English system of which it was in most respects an imitation – had grafted on to it in 1851 provision for appointing local general medical practitioners (GPs) to work outside the workhouse walls. A dispensary medical service was provided whereby, within each of the more than 700 districts into which the country was divided, a salaried medical officer could be consulted by a sick person, having obtained from a Poor Law guardian a 'ticket' which attested to inability to pay for a doctor's services. In essentials this system stayed in place until the early 1970s. The General Medical Service (GMS) arrangements, which then superseded the dispensaries, modified the old system by giving the patient a choice of doctor after having been subjected to a more systematic and nationally uniform regime of means testing.

Some glaring absences may have been as important as other looming presences. Here, Barrington points up how the relative weakness of the labour movement, of socialist ideas and of friendly societies left only the state acting as a mediating party between doctor and patient. The exclusion of Ireland from the Medical Benefit of the 1911 National Insurance Act – which for British insured workers met the cost of GP consultations and prescribed medicines – was crucial here. By the late 1930s half of the British adult population attended a GP free of charge under National Insurance entitlements (Digby and Bosanquet, 1988). In Ireland free GP attendance sustained by state-channelled funding was still available only through the dispensary service from which the Poor Law's name had been removed. It was now called Public Assistance. Ireland's exclusion from medical benefit under the National Insurance Act 1911 was taken up by the Irish Trade Union Congress (ITUC). However, as the ITUC's annual report for 1912 makes clear, trade union protests to the Irish Parliamentary Party – which had moved the amendment to exclude Ireland from the medical benefit – carried little weight compared with the views of the Catholic bishops and the doctors. Although the scope of coverage provided by the state insurance scheme differed between Britain and Ireland, the near-fatal undermining of the previously expanding friendly society movement was to be a feature of its operation in both countries. A badge of working class respect-ability and self-sufficiency, friendly society membership in its period of strength had had significant quality of medical service implications: 'whereas a patient had to accept whatever the dispensary doctor offered him in treatment or courtesy, a friendly society doctor had to meet often exacting standards which the society could set, or run the risk of being replaced' (Buckley, 1987: 48).

By 1911 a measure granting Home Rule to Ireland was expected soon to become law. The influential Irish opposition at its initiation to the whole state insurance scheme (which covered the contingencies of unemployment as well as those of health) reflected fears that social legislation of this kind would leave a Home Rule government with a level of expenditure much in excess of its revenue. Such legislation was designed for a predominantly industrial Britain rather than a predominantly agricultural Ireland, its opponents maintained. The less developed country could not afford to adopt the 'champagne standard of living' that was within the means of its more developed neighbour. The idea that social legislation and the rights it conferred should bear the brunt of bringing the budget into balance was, however, far from enjoying universal acceptance,. Nor did a taste for champagne (if such it was) disappear under self-government. As Barrington (1987: 283) notes, events in Britain, such as the appearance of the Beveridge Report and the creation of the National Health Service during the 1940s, had 'immense' indirect effects in Ireland. Ongoing interaction between the two states through a variety of different channels stimulated demands for a health service 'arguably beyond the means of a country at Ireland's level of development'.

With less territory but more independent decision-making power than Ireland was envisaged as having under Home Rule, the Irish Free State under Cumann na nGaedheal rule in the 1920s sought to reduce social spending in order to promote the competitiveness of Irish agricultural goods in the British market. Fianna Fáil's advent to power in 1932 led to a switch to protectionism in economic policy, accompanied by a more active concern with social protection in the health, housing and social welfare fields. But even before this switch was made, a remarkable means of evading the constraints imposed by relative underdevelopment on the funding of health services had been devised – the Irish Hospitals Sweepstake.

The Sweepstake had its origins in the financial crisis being experienced by voluntary hospitals. By 1930, lobbying on behalf of some of these hospitals had led to legislation that allowed a sweepstake to be organised for their benefit. The triumvirate of Richard Duggan, Joseph McGrath and Spencer Freeman undertook this organisation. Under their direction the Irish Hospitals Sweepstake was to generate cash in a manner that surpassed all initial expectations, for distribution by the government among the public as well as the voluntary hospitals. Most of this money was raised by the sale of tickets outside Ireland. Initially, Britain provided the main market for sales. But new legal restrictions, which choked off promotional publicity, together with the rising popularity of the football pools, led to the USA becoming the major consumer of tickets and provider of funds in the years after the Second World War. The launching of state lotteries by an increasing number of US states eventually pushed the Irish Hospitals Sweepstake into decline: the decision in the mid-1980s to launch an

Irish National Lottery and to place its management in the hands of An Post brought its era to a close. While health activities and organisations feature among the range of the National Lottery's beneficiaries, the largesse of the Hospitals Sweepstake was solely confined to hospital funding. Ironically, as a gaming-centred history of the enterprise noted, 'the rain of pound notes from the Irish Sweep which saved Ireland's hospitals in dire emergency has in some ways made the problem of caring for the nation's sick not easier but more difficult' (Webb, 1968: 82). A profusion of Sweepstake proceeds allowed the difficult issue of rationalising hospital provision to be avoided at the same time as a high level of capital investment spread across the excessive number of existing and some new hospitals was sowing the seeds of an onerous current spending requirement. This was a tab the more prosaic forms of public funding such as taxation and borrowing would subsequently have to pick up.

In the independent Irish state's large and ubiquitously influential (Chubb, 1992: 3–7) neighbour, the United Kingdom, what public expenditure on health underpinned by the end of the 1940s was an attempt to realise Sir William Beveridge's model of a service 'providing full preventive and curative treatment of every kind to every citizen without exceptions, without a remuneration limit and without an economic barrier at any point to delay recourse to it'. When the Beveridge Report was published in 1942, it generated an enormous public response among a population mobilised for the prosecution of a 'total' war:

> His proposals were to take on vast symbolic significance as they came to be seen as a 'preview' of the post-war British 'dream'. The Beveridge Report was to become the best-selling bureaucratic memo in British history (over half a million copies were purchased). The fervour with which it was received clearly reflected a deep societal appetite for wide-scale social reform. (Hay, 1996: 29)

The independent Irish state's experience of an 'Emergency' was a very different one. Here the end of the World War tended to be seen less as an opportunity to begin building the New Jerusalem than as a change from one set of trepidation-inducing difficulties and threats to another (see, for instance, Wolf, 1996). The unveiling of Beveridge's national health service model stimulated discussion of the need to reform Irish health service provision but, rather than producing a high degree of consensus as in Britain, the Irish health service reform question became surrounded by deepening conflict. The Beveridge-influenced plans for gradually increasing state involvement in the provision of services free of user charge to all that emanated first from the Department of Local Government and Public Health and then, after 1947, from the Department of Health, encountered strong opposition from a powerful alliance of the Catholic Church hierarchy and the medical profession. These opponents argued that a narrowly restricted role for free-to-user services, whose supply was directly controlled by the state, was all that could be reconciled with the key principle of subsidiarity enshrined in Catholic social teaching (Whyte, 1980; Barrington, 1987)

The resolution of this conflict over health service reform involving state, medical profession and church reaffirmed moralism, means-testing and private medical practice. Catholic girls and women were not safe, the bishops felt, at the time of the 1950–1 Mother and Child scheme proposals, in the hands of state medical officials who might not anathematise 'birth limitation and abortion' in the desired fashion. Thereafter, with regard to the maintenance of Catholic ethical standards in medical practice, the church and a medical profession, which had enjoyed invaluable episcopal support in limiting the socialisation of medicine, continued, Barrington argues, to sustain an effective alliance. Because of this, restricted availability of family planning services, sterilisation procedures and infertility treatments remains a feature of today's Irish health care system. Means testing was confirmed as a basic feature of the publicly provided services by the 1953 Health Act which defined three categories of service-users with entitlements to receive free services, shrinking as level of income rose. Thus, a stratification which put about 35 per cent of the population in a low income category, about 50 per cent in a middle income one and about 15 per cent in a higher income one, came into being. This remained in place until 1991 when the upper-income and middle-income categories were merged on the basis of the middle income group's entitlements. Today, possessing a medical card (being in the lower income Category I) gives access to all publicly provided services free of charge. The principal user charges which members of the merged higher income category (Category II) must pay are levied for GP visits, drug prescriptions, visits to hospital outpatient departments and accommodation in a public hospital.

The third, upper income, category created in 1953 may have vanished from the scene but an important legacy of its creation lingers on. Public policy encouragement of private insurance cover for hospital accommodation and treatment being acquired by those with minimal eligibility to use public services without charge was expressed through the creation of the state-sponsored Voluntary Health Insurance Board (VHI) in 1957 and through the availability to subscribers of income tax relief on their VHI premiums. Those needing private cover because of minimal public entitlements made up a proportion of the population deliberately maintained around the 15 per cent mark but by the time this third category was abolished the population proportion with VHI cover was about twice as large.

The relationship between public and private medicine in Ireland is, Nolan (1991: 22) points out, 'not one between two separate parallel systems: rather the private and public elements are intertwined'. The manner in which the mid-century conflict over health service reform was defused created the conditions for this 'extraordinary symbiosis of public and private medicine' (Barrington,

1987: 285). The complex public/private mix thus created effectively defines a
new three-way stratification of the state's population with regard to health
service access. These three distinct categories are:

1   Those with medical cards who have public services free of charge but, with
    very few exceptions, have no insurance cover and therefore no effective
    access to hospital services on a private basis.
2   Those without medical cards and without insurance cover who are subject
    to user charges for GPs, prescribed drugs and public hospital usage and have
    no effective access to hospital services on a private basis.
3   Those without medical cards and with insurance cover who incur GP,
    prescribed drugs and public hospital user charges and have effective access
    to hospital services on a private basis.

The 1950s thus emerge as the period in which access and entitlement
differentials that continue to be a central feature of Irish health care provision
were put in place. Apart from the ending of the dispensary doctor system in the
early 1970s, the most important changes to take place in the system since that
decade have concerned the centralisation of financing and the regionalisation
of administration. Once financed through a combination of local government
rate revenue and central government grants, the funding of the public health
services by stages became solely the responsibility of central government during
the 1960s and 1970s. Linked to the removal of funding responsibility from local
authorities was the removal of their service delivery role. Around thirty counties
and county boroughs gave way after 1970 to eight regional health boards.
Service-providing professionals were strongly represented on these boards
alongside elected local authority members, while the services themselves were
organised within a three 'programme' management structure recommended by
the consultants, McKinsey & Company. This sub-divided provision into general
hospital care, special hospital care (for psychiatric patients or the mentally
handicapped) and community care (for details, see Hensey, 1988).

Summarising the specific nature of the Irish health care system, we can say
that the legacy of British rule, the policies of post-independence governments
of different party composition, the power of the Catholic Church and the
influence of the medical profession have interacted to produce a complicated
mix of private and public health care provision. The private element has been
publicly subsidised in a variety of ways. The public element is marked by the
combination of centralised funding with regionalised delivery. How this system
came under sustained criticism for its cost, its imbalances and its inequities after
its completion in the 1970s is examined next.

Changes in service provision

The completion of the Irish health care system's construction coincided with the advent of insistent international calls for the radical reorientation of the type of service provision structure it exemplified. The major components of this envisaged reorientation have been a shift in emphasis from curative to preventive interventions and the priority given to primary health care provision rather than the secondary or tertiary levels of the health care system.

The rationale for an enhanced role for prevention stems from the dominance of chronic diseases like cancer and heart disease within the present day pattern of ill-health. The risk of developing these diseases is widely agreed to be related to how people live their everyday lives – to the diet they eat, to whether or not they take exercise, to cigarette smoking. Many premature deaths and episodes of serious illness could therefore be prevented by changes in currently prevailing lifestyles. Developing the provision of health care at the primary level has, since the Declaration of the World Health Assembly at Alma Ata in 1978, been seen as the means by which available resources can be used as effectively and efficiently as possible to address the major health needs of the population. Embracing inter-sectoral collaboration and community participation, the primary health care concept ranges much more widely than the field of health services as conventionally defined. Within that field, it is associated with maximising the provision of services within local community, as opposed to large institutional settings.

Clearly, given the role of organisations like the World Health Organisation (WHO) in pushing reorientation up the policy agenda, the impetus for change was coming in part from within the professional world of medicine. But forces external to that world were also playing a significant part. As Nettleton (1995: 5) observes, 'during the last two decades the institution of medicine and the biomedical model have increasingly been challenged by critiques emerging from both popular and academic sources. These criticisms have been intensified within the context of the escalating costs of health care.'

Within the Irish context, cost containment concerns were clearly to the fore in the case of the Working Party on the General Medical Service (1984). This Working Party, consisting of Department of Health officials, regional Health Board managers and doctors' representatives reviewed the first decade of operation of this scheme which had provided free GP visits and drug prescriptions to Category I members since 1972 with freedom of choice of doctor for the eligible patient and fee-for-item-of-service remuneration for the participating doctor. The Working Party fully endorsed the concept and extensively deployed the rhetoric of WHO's primary health care, but what the actual content of its proposals mirrored was the kind of changes that had taken place in Britain since the introduction there in 1965 of the GPs' Charter. Thus, its Report advocated financial incentives to GPs for the formation of group practices and the provision of out-of-hours cover; grants for the improvement of practice premises; the attachment to or grant-aided employment by practices of ancillary staff (principally nurses) and the provision of access to hospital facilities for GPs. The cost-containing *quid pro quo* sought from the doctors was modification of the existing fee-for-item-of-service remuneration arrangement and co-operation with a scheme of target drug costs per Category I patient. That the review was an exercise in interest group bargaining as much as policy analysis was made clear by the manner in which maintenance of the patient population's existing eligibility stratification was assumed from the outset of the discussion.

The following year, 1985, saw a wider-ranging and more detached appraisal of the Irish health care system's performance, with more radical proposals for change being put forward by a health economist, A. Dale Tussing. The basic problem, according to his analysis, was that the incentive structure identifiable within the Irish health care system encouraged wasteful resource over-use. The solution to this problem lay in reorganising the system so that incentives to economise were put in place both for providers and consumers. International experience indicated that either market or non-market mechanisms could provide the basis of a strategy to achieve such a reorganisation over the medium to long term. Compatible with either strategic choice were a number of reforms whose immediate adoption was advocated by Tussing. First, an incentive-prompted shift towards lower cost primary care could be brought about by introducing free GP care for all, with capitation-based payment to the GPs while at the same time introducing charges on middle and higher income (Categories II and III) patients for hospital services that had hitherto been free. Second, all forms of public subsidy to private care usage should cease. Third, more emphasis should be put on quality assurance, experimental innovation and addressing the weakly developed state of general practice (with incentives for GPs to form group practices, employ 'physician auxiliaries' etc.). Fourth, there should be better resourcing of dentistry, of health education and of research and analysis from a health economics and/or social policy perspective.

While the Working Party and Tussing differed significantly as regards detailed proposals (particularly regarding free service eligibility for patients and remuneration arrangements for doctors), both reflected international thinking on the need for system reorientation in their calls for a shift in emphasis towards primary care and preventive intervention. A tendency to conflate the concept of primary care with the medical institution of general practice in a way that marginalises the contribution of the Health Board Community Care programmes to the provision of primary care was also common to both, however. This imbalance within the health policy analysis literature was redressed by the comprehensive overview of the community care programme services published by the National Economic and Social Council (NESC) in

1987. It noted the glaring contrast between official statements that care in the community was a desirable objective and an observed lack of commitment 'to specify the implications of this goal in terms of the services necessary to make it a reality' and a failure to allocate resources to support the development of this range of services. NESC highlighted the inadequacy of the information available for the planning and evaluation of community care services and the manner in which organisational problems, inter-professional rivalries and the separation of medical general practice from the other forms of primary care provided in the community context hampered service development. The consequences of the gap between the rhetoric of community care and its reality were also graphically highlighted by an important study of the carers of dependent elderly people carried out for the National Council for the Aged (O'Connor and Ruddle, 1988; see also Blackwell et al., 1992).

The acceptance within Irish policy discussion of the case being made internationally for system reorientation also found expression during the mid-1980s in the Department of Health's 1986 consultative statement *Health – The Wider Dimensions* and in the 1987 report of an expert working group set up by the Health Education Bureau, *Promoting Health Through Public Policy* (Health Education Bureau, 1987). Shifting emphasis on to prevention had long been recognised as requiring much greater provision of health education. Now the terms in which health education had hitherto been conceived were giving way to a more radical concept – that of health promotion. This envisaged adding supportive environmental interventions to the existing emphasis on developing the life skills and competencies of the individual in order 'to make the healthier choice the easier choice'. The aspiration that health concerns should become a major consideration across all sectors of societal activity at international, national and local levels runs through these documents. Ironically, the overriding political concern to emerge in Ireland at this time was that immediate action be taken to reduce the heavy burden of debt that a decade of state borrowing to fund current expenditure deficits had created. The across-the-board cuts in expenditure through which this end was pursued towards the end of the 1980s did not spare the costly health care system. From this period also date the user charges for hospital accommodation and outpatient visits to which those outside Category I continue to be subject.

Management of services

Retrenchment and new user-charging provided the context within which the Commission on Health Funding set about reviewing the equity, comprehensiveness and cost-effectiveness of Irish service provision. The existing tax-based funding system was favoured in its 1989 report and 'the kernel of the

Commission's conclusions is that the solution to the problem facing the Irish health services does not lie primarily in the system of funding but rather in the way that services are planned, organised and delivered' (Commission on Health Funding, 1989, para. 2.45). Services needed to be managed rather than the existing situation of being administered. Accountability for performance, financial incentive to perform and management training were the features distinguishing the desired manager from the existing administrator. A new structure for management culture and practice to develop within was to be pro-vided by creating a new Health Services Executive Authority that would replace the existing health boards and take responsibility for the delivery of 'a core level of publicly-funded services'. Apart from the merging of the middle and higher income categories, the existing eligibility stratification for public services was to be retained. On grounds of equity, and in the light of the uncertain future the VHI system faced with the advent of a competitive single European market in 1992, the Commission advocated changes in the public/private mix – principally the gradual elimination of all public subsidies to private care and the creation of 'a common waiting list for both public and private patients, from which cases would be taken in order of medically established priority'. The boundary between 'core' services to be supported by public funding and peripheral ones whose full economic cost would presumably fall on the private resources of individual users was delineated only in very broad terms by the Report, leaving unclear what the full practical implications of this key distinction might be.

By the end of the 1980s considerable analysis of the Irish health care system had taken place. The extent to which the introduction of policy change in the 1990s has or has not been prompted by the criticisms made is the focus of this paper's concluding section.

Policy change in the 1990s

By the end of the 1990s the broad context within which discussion of policy issues relating to health and health care took place was considerably different from that prevailing at the end of the 1980s. The 'Celtic Tiger' economy displayed a buoyancy scarcely imaginable a decade earlier, the public finances were in much better shape and expenditure retrenchment had given way to resumed expenditure growth (Wiley, 1997; 1998). Within this context, the health care access and entitlement differentials defined in the 1950s survived intact to a remarkable degree. The merger of Categories II and III did alter the eligibility stratification pattern. But stringently means-tested access to Category I had not diminished substantially. The only significant changes in this regard were, first, that everyone over seventy years of age became eligible for a medical card regardless of their income in 2001 and, second, that some younger people moving from unemployment into employment have since the mid-1990s been allowed to retain their medical cards even if their income puts them over the qualifying limit for a fixed transitional period of time.[1]

In relation to the public/private mix, the Commission on Health Funding's common waiting list recommendation was not acted upon. Instead, the Programme for Economic and Social Progress agreed between the social partners in 1991 provided for the phasing in of a new system whereby private patients in public hospitals would be accommodated only in private or semi-private beds, with the designation of all beds as private or public being completed over the phasing-in period. The Commission on Health Funding had estimated that with tax relief on premiums ended, common waiting lists and an erosion 'after 1992' of community rating (that is, the same premiums for all subscribers regardless of age or risk, see Light, chapter 4 below) had opened up the market and ended the VHI monopoly, the number of people with private insurance could fall by a third. On the basis of survey data showing nearly two thirds of insured respondents opting for 'being sure of getting into hospital quickly when you need treatment' as their 'most important' reason for having VHI cover, Nolan (1991) suggested that this could turn out to be an underestimate. In practice, premiums have risen as health care inflation considerably outstrips overall inflation within the economy and the value of the tax relief available has been curtailed rather than eliminated. Yet, towards the end of 1990s, the demand for health insurance appears as buoyant as ever in a context where European Union competition law has to date meant the virtual monopoly of VHI turning into a duopoly with the entry into the market of the British company, BUPA. The speed and certainty of hospital access differential between private and public patients has been much criticised but it plainly remains a key feature of the operation of the Irish health care system.

In the case of the principal early 1970s additions to the system – the GMS and the health boards – a somewhat greater degree of change has occurred or is in the offing. Payment for GMS doctors changed from a fee-for-service to a capitation base by negotiated agreement in 1989, thus removing a major incentive to resource overuse indicted by Tussing (1985). This change was linked to the provision of funding for doctors to employ ancillary staff (such as secretaries and nurses) and to improve their practice premises and equipment. New General Practice Unit support structures were also installed at Department of Health and regional health board levels. Drug expenditure growth has been tackled by both setting an overall target and giving each doctor an individualised drug budget target. Savings made provide a source of ongoing funding for general practice development. The annual rate of growth of drugs spending fell after this scheme went into operation but there is a danger that it could change

1   Editor's note. In late 2004 the government announced proposals to increase the number of medical cardholders by 230,000 from 1 January 2005 – see Curry, chapter 1 above.

doctors' prescribing behaviour in ways that reinvent the two-tier system the GMS was designed to get rid of by, for example, leading to a lower rate of introduction of (expensive) new drugs among medical card patients as compared with fee-paying patients (Murphy, 1997).

The abolition of the health boards recommended by the Commission on Health Funding has not taken place.[2] Indeed, changes affecting the organisation of services in the Eastern Region – where the existing regional board has been replaced by three 'area' boards and a regional authority – have meant that there are now more of these bodies in existence than ever before. There has, however, been an attempt to change the way in which they perform. In broad terms the changes introduced have been intended to foster a managerial rather than an administrative culture, as advocated by the Commission on Health Funding (1989). In particular, the Boards (and the new Eastern Regional Health Authority) have begun to deal directly, through a service contract system based on performance specification and accountability, with large voluntary hospitals which are owned and controlled by Catholic religious orders or other interests of a religious denominational character. The manner in which these hospitals had previously engaged in national level budget negotiation with the Department of Health had weakened regional management of services since its inception in the early 1970s. If, as intended, its scope is gradually extended, this change should have its greatest impact on service delivery in the Eastern region, which contains nearly a third of the state's population and where hospitals of this type have historically been major service providers and resource users. Time will tell if the envisaged ending of chronic service fragmentation in the Eastern region rather than simply the addition of a further layer of unproductive bureaucracy results from the changes being made.

The late 1980s retrenchment witnessed, among other things, the demise of the Health Education Bureau and its replacement by a new national Health Promotion structure. With a Cabinet sub-committee at its apex, a dedicated unit within the Department of Health as its executive engine, a Chair in Health Promotion in the National University of Ireland, Galway to stimulate supportive research and teaching as well as a new range of advisory body inputs, this structure looked impressive on paper. In reality, however, an ambitious and expansive policy concept was being endorsed at a time when the real level of resources available to develop and set it in operation were being contracted. A national teacher education programme developed by the Health Education Bureau was discontinued while some regional health boards reacted to reduced budgets by scrapping virtually all their health education/health promotion activity.

2   Editor's note. Subsequent to the completion of this chapter the Irish government announced radical reforms in the health service, including the abolition of the health boards (See McCluskey, chapter 15 below). The general thrust of the final section of Murray's paper would appear to presage such developments but their introduction has occurred much sooner than he might have anticipated.

A renewed, and more concrete, emphasis within Irish health policy on the role health promotion could play in generating 'health gain' was provided by the goals and targets of the national health strategy statement *Shaping a Healthier Future* (Department of Health, 1994a). Here, increased Irish life expectancy was conceived as the end point of a mobilisation of effort which focused on the main causes of premature mortality – heart disease and cancer – and the risk factors associated with these diseases: smoking, alcohol, nutrition and diet, exercise, cholesterol and blood pressure. However, definite commitments of additional resources for supportive action programmes did not accompany the goal and target setting exercises, some of the targets were nor properly quantified and arrangements for monitoring progress – or the lack of it – towards target achievement were only belatedly addressed. When evidence became available in the late 1990s that risk factor reduction targets were clearly not on the way to being met, the official response was extraordinarily muted. As noted above, health promotion is supposed to add to health education the provision of environmental supports for styles of life that enhance or maintain health. But, apart from increased restriction of smoking and of tobacco product promotion, no environmental changes are being introduced. The successful achievement of the targets set is reliant instead on the widespread adoption of a healthier lifestyle within the population in response to the stimulus of interpersonal and mass media communication campaigns. Thus, with the important exception of smoking, health promotion is being talked about by policy makers but what they are enacting is, in essence, still health education.

Conclusion

If a connecting thread runs through the 1990s mix of status quo maintenance and new departures that have just been described, it is the adoption by the health care system's policy makers of a strategic management approach. Strategic management is an invention of the world of business enterprises. A key emphasis in the business history literature is the manner in which structure follows strategy, with the organisation adapting itself to the nature of the tasks it performs (Chandler, 1962). Led off by *Shaping a Healthier Future*, management strategy statements relating to Irish health care have proliferated while structural change of limited scope has been slowly implemented within the system to which they refer.

A resurgent interest in the scholarly analysis of Irish health policy issues is evident in recent years (*Administration*, various years; O'Donovan and Casey, 1995: Cleary and Treacy, 1997; Robins, 1997; Wiley, 1997; Leahy and Wiley, 1998; McAuliffe and Joyce, 1998; O'Carroll, 1998). Health has also become a high profile area of political controversy with rival party proposals for change very much to the fore in the general election campaign of 2002. At this election a large cohort of Independents whose campaigns were primarily focused on particular, localised perceived shortcomings of the health care system were returned to the Dáil. With health expenditure now rising at a rate that can hardly be sustained (Wiley, 2002) and public dissatisfaction with the services being provided remaining unassuaged, it is safe to forecast that we will have much discussion of health care reform in Ireland over the next few years. But the extent to which such discussion is accompanied by action, or the shape this action may take, are not so easy to predict.

Chapter 4

Making competition fair for health insurance in Ireland

Donald W. Light

Modern medicine is a major domain of applied science and technology, but infused with values so that it appears to be more rational than it is (Payer, 1988). This is an irony of many 'rational' systems that in fact differ from culture to culture (and subculture to subculture), which Dobbin (1994) calls 'instrumentally rational cultural systems'. As it applies science and technology in culturally shaped ways, medicine is also surrounded by risk and uncertainty. The risks involved are not only clinical, around which states have developed a complex set of regulations, but financial as well. The sickest two per cent of a population need such intensive and extensive care that they consume 41 per cent of all costs (Berk and Monheit, 1992), and to make matters worse, considerable variability surrounds this highly skewed distribution. You never can tell with these very sick patients what will go wrong next (or what sudden improvement will occur); so you cannot tell how much they will cost.

As high-tech modern medicine created these huge differences in cost, many industrialised countries (except the United States) established one kind or another of universal health insurance or access to services as an essential service and a right of residency. Most of these systems for providing universal access to needed health care services do not allow competition, because fair competition is extremely difficult to arrange in health insurance. Competition, as Adam Smith observed in the eighteenth century, can benefit society only if markets have a number of structural characteristics that channel competitive energies towards providing better value, greater efficiency, and better service (Rice, 1998; Light, 1999). Otherwise, competitors make society worse through collusion, cream-skimming, and other techniques that exploit customers and the rest of society. Medicine and health insurance markets have almost none of these structural characteristics that protect policyholders and patients from being exploited. For example, there are almost never many sellers and full market information about price, quality and service – two of ten requirements for competition to benefit rather than harm society. People who become ill, injured, or disabled do not meet those conditions for beneficial competition, because they are vulnerable, usually unable to shop, and relatively uninformed about the highly technical choices that must be made. Instead, there are usually only one, two or three insurance companies and not very complete or accessible information on how their policies and service compare with each other. Insurance companies can make money much more easily by selectively marketing to healthier consumers and by discriminating directly or indirectly against people with health problems or risks than by becoming more efficient. Many of the techniques are described in an earlier article (Light, 1992). Just by avoiding some of the very ill, or by getting them to drop out by serving them badly, an insurance company can make millions in profits.

Despite these problems, American policy makers and consulting firms have been vigorously exporting to European nations and many developing countries since the 1980s the idea that competitive health insurance will slow down or lower health care costs. However, for reasons explained below, it is nearly impossible to construct equitable markets in health insurance that reward efficiency and services, rather than discriminating against the sick and those at high risk. Many countries have concluded that competition between *providers* might save money, but a uniform means of collecting premiums or taxes is cheaper and more equitable than having competing insurers design a range of health insurance policies, market them, and collect the premiums (Cherichovsky, 1995).

These reservations notwithstanding, the European Union issued a directive in 1992 that required all nations to introduce competition among health insurers, while preserving the 'social good' of each country. Given that such competition (for reasons explained below) challenges the values and culture of any nation with universal health care (which is all of Europe), this seemingly straightforward directive to foster 'economic vitality' and 'efficiency' challenges the solidarity and deeply held values about family and community of nations like Ireland.

All societies decide how much risk and of what kind various parties can bear and what remedies are to be made available. There are no 'free markets'. Competitors cannot compete over anything using any tactic. For example, you cannot save money by taking your chances with a discount airline that inspects its planes only half as often as is deemed safe. Nor can you buy uninspected food for half price, even if you are poor. Why? Because through experience (and often tragedies), societies decide that unsafe planes and contaminated food contain too many hidden risks that customers cannot detect, and that could harm or kill them. Conversely, many markets with inferior products are not regulated nearly as much, like audio equipment, because people's lives are not endangered and they can obtain good market information about how different systems perform. Thus states construct, in Dobbin's (1994) wonderfully ironic term, markets as 'instrumentally rational cultural systems'.

The case of Ireland: reluctant universalism

Nations vary in their culture and motives for establishing health care systems and shaping them as they do. Until the 1950s, the Republic of Ireland had provided free care only for the poor, through the poor laws and subsequently local boards and then county boards (Curry, 1993). The non-poor paid private fees. Free services for the poor and no government provision otherwise are a rather minimal, tough approach that is particularly hard on the working class. It usually means that working-class and even middle-class patients are forced to use up their life's savings and be driven into poverty if they have a serious medical problem. As the post-war cost of hospital-based care and medical technology rose sharply, the government began to think out how it could make health care accessible to everyone yet affordable. It granted limited eligibility in 1953 for free hospital services and established the Voluntary Health Insurance Board (VHI) in 1957 as a non-profit, semi-state but independent body that offered hospital-based insurance to those not eligible for free care.

VHI policies were based on three principles: community rating (the same premiums for all subscribers regardless of age or risk), open enrolment, and lifetime coverage. Thus, like early Blue Cross legislation in the US, Irish leaders decided to provide non-profit voluntary health insurance. But unlike the US, they set their cultural boundaries as follows: that the working and middle classes needed better financial access to medical services and that this should happen, not through a national service as in the United Kingdom but through private services reimbursed by equitable, non-profit, state-sponsored health insurance that guaranteed open enrolment, community rating and lifetime coverage (if one could afford to continue to pay the premiums). VHI, in conjunction with health services for the poor, could therefore be considered one form of an institutionally rational but culturally shaped health insurance system.

In 1991, the costly hospital-based services were extended free to everyone, another tough-minded decision about the amount of financial burden and risk that citizens should bear. Many other countries had long since provided universal access to hospital and non-hospital services. Primary-care services remained free only to the 35 per cent of the population eligible for low-income medical cards. Thus as a social institution, VHI evolved from a voluntary, non-profit, community-rated way for the non-poor to cover their risk for the costs of hospital-based services, to a supplementary policy that bought quicker access and upgraded services in specialty and hospital care, backed by a national health service.

These recent changes reflect a certain cultural ambiguity, namely state-legitimated two-tier health care, yet carefully protected from the exploitations of risk-rated private health insurance (Light, 1992). In terms of equity, this arrangement is less equitable than a system like Sweden's that aimed from the start to offer universal access to a health care system so good that no one would want to take out private insurance. But as a non-profit, community-rated upgrade it is far more equitable than risk-rated private insurance and the upgrades that are found in many countries such as Great Britain, because the Irish system does not allow insurers to single out the most profitable procedures, disorders or subscribers from the national service or system. Moreover, among all the gradations of what 'community rating' can mean – from American-style 'community rating' that actually targets selected groups with bands and ranges (Orwellian newspeak for mild risk rating), to community rating a large population – VHI policies offer the same rate nationwide for each of five policies that have very similar coverages and differ largely in the degree of private care they offer (VHI, 1996).

Coverage has focused heavily on queue-jumping the waiting lists in the public system for elective surgical and specialty procedures, on better accommodation (semi-private or private rooms, in public or private hospitals) and on choice of consultant. Premiums are remarkably low by international standards, though the Irish constantly complain about how expensive they are and fume whenever there is a small increase. In 1996, the tax-deductible premiums for an individual subscribing to the most popular Plan B cost about the same after taxes as a weekend holiday for two at a hotel in Dublin. About 40 per cent of the population have chosen to buy VHI policies. In my judgement, Irish private health insurance is about as equitable and affordable as health insurance can be and still provide a two-tier upgrade for the middle classes.

American analysts might well predict that private-insurance upgrades of a national health service would siphon off middle-class support for the public system, causing it to deteriorate into a welfare system with the low level of care that existed under the nineteenth-century poor laws and dispensaries. So far, however, the national service seems to be considered as reasonably good, though slow to do elective investigations or procedures, and as having become steadily better over the past several years. At the same time, the public system has become dependent on the VHI upgrades to induce a large minority of the population to pay for most of their medical care above and beyond what they pay for the public system through taxes.

Making competition fair

After the 1992 EU directive, the Dáil set about drafting an act designed to foster competitive health insurance within an equitable framework that would preserve the cultural repertoire (almost a mantra) of community rating, open enrolment, and lifetime coverage (Health Insurance Act 1994). The particulars of the 1994 Act, however, were drafted imperfectly by staff who appear not to have appreciated the range and subtlety of risk-rating techniques that commercial insurers can use. As a result, a clever insurer could find ways to design risk-rated policies and get them registered.

Given that the sickest two per cent of a large pool consume on average 41 per cent of the total medical expenditures, and the sickest 10 per cent consume 72 per cent (Berk and Monheit, 1992), competing insurers can make much larger profits more easily by taking in fewer than their proportionate share of these sick people, or by inducing them to dis-enrol, than by becoming more efficient or providing better service. Increasing operational efficiency or improving service is hard work; risk selection is not. Unless careful safeguards are put in place, competition between health insurers obeys the Inverse Coverage Law (Light, 1992): the more people need insurance, the less coverage they will get and the more they will pay for what they get. Such medical needs strongly correlate with age and relative poverty.

In theory, this basic problem of inequality in risks could be solved by adjusting the revenue to insurance pools by risk so that it would match their expenditures. Otherwise, insurers with a larger proportion of healthier subscribers would make handsome profits, and insurers with a larger proportion of sicker subscribers would suffer substantial losses. But extensive research to identify risk adjusters that might prevent such adverse selection in competition between health insurers has found that the 'maximum explainable variance in annual acute health care expenditures per individual is around 15 per cent', leaving at least 85 per cent open to cream-skimming (van de Ven and van Vliet, 1992). Worse, even if risk adjusters were used, there are many ways for an insurer to select good risks anyway. There are direct forms of risk rating, such as denying coverage for cardiac conditions or charging a higher premium, and indirect methods, such as policy design and marketing. Some techniques are front-end, such as those just mentioned, and some are back-end, such as de-selecting higher risks by aggravating procedures, delaying or obstructing access, and limiting extended treatments (Light, 1992). For these and other reasons, having competition in health insurance that benefits society by lowering costs and improving services, rather than through discrimination, is difficult to attain. This observation illustrates a more fundamental point about neoclassical economics and the radical assertion of Adam Smith, that society can actually benefit from everyone pursuing their self-interests, but only if an extensive set of conditions exist (Enthoven, 1988; Light, 1994). Otherwise, competition will harm society in a number of ways, as competitors exploit customers and/or the state.

It took until 1996 to develop the regulations of the Act (Statutory Instruments, 1996), but soon afterwards one of Europe's largest health insurers launched a marketing blitz for Ireland's first age-graded policies. The next day, 2,500 callers rang its tele-sales centre for applications, and some of the press dutifully published its press materials without critical review (Seekamp, 1996). What the British Union Provident Association (BUPA) offered were policies apparently designed to compete head-to-head with each of VHI's five policies. But while the basic policy was community rated, the premiums for the upgrades were age-graded. Because they paid cash instead of upgraded services, these 'cash plans' were said by BUPA not to be technically 'insurance' and therefore not covered by the Health Insurance Act of 1994.

If one compared the after-tax group premiums of VHI's most popular Plan B to BUPA's competing policy, BUPA's premiums were 10 per cent lower for subscribers under 19, four per cent lower for subscribers 19 to 49, 20 per cent higher for people 50 to 54, and 28 per cent higher for those over 54. BUPA apparently intended to compete, not primarily by being more efficient or providing better service, but by drawing off younger subscribers from VHI. Moreover, this competition among insurers was not aimed at addressing the real sources of waste in the underlying hospital-centred delivery system.

These realities raise basic questions about whether the European Union was clear about what it wanted to accomplish with its directive to have insurer competition, as distinct from provider competition. VHI was already a very efficient insurer, spending only two per cent of premiums on administration compared to about 12 per cent for commercial insurers. Is this a case where, as Europe's leading expert on risk rating and health insurance writes, '*efficient* insurers might be driven out of the market by *inefficient* insurers who are successful in cream-skimming . . . so there is no social gain . . . [but] only social welfare loses'? (van de Ven, 1991: 438). Moreover, because VHI with its social rather than commercial ethos had paid out almost all premiums for patient care, it had not built up a surplus or reserves. BUPA, reflecting a commercial ethos, paid out significantly less and had accumulated nearly $1 billion in reserves. Thus, BUPA could sustain losses for years, while any significant shift of younger subscribers would quickly drive VHI towards bankruptcy unless it started to risk rate as well.

Behind risk- and community-rating are two different theories of justice and fairness, each embodying a different value set (Daniels, 1985; 1988; Light, 1992). The theory of actuarial fairness holds that it is unfair to make those who are healthier subsidise those who are sicker or at higher risk. It rests on a libertarian philosophy that fiercely defends (negative) rights for individuals (Nozick, 1974). For example, to take an easy case like smoking, a libertarian would ask, 'Why should *my* premium go to pay in part for the consequences of *their* behaviour? If they want to smoke, let them pay for their higher risk.' But other factors complicate this position. For example, smoking is heavily induced by advertising and becomes addictive; so how voluntary is it? Also, how much more should the smokers' premia be to reflect *fairly* their higher risk? The answers get very, perhaps impossibly, complicated, which then raises the question of whether actuarial fairness can be done fairly.[1] In addition, the same libertarian philosophy would apply to diabetes, asthma, heart disease and old age: 'Why should *my* premium go in part to pay for *their* problems?' Another problem is that risk-rating, especially in competitive markets, elaborates on itself, so that finer and finer distinctions get made. The more precise it becomes, the less of an insurance function occurs, until each risk group is essentially prepaying its own risk. For example, diabetic women age 60 to 64 with a family history of heart disease would pay their 'actuarially fair' premium, while diabetic women 55 to 59 with a family history of heart disease would pay theirs. Relative poverty is a major predictor of all health problems, so that these triple-risk women would have to pay still higher premia as their incomes decline.

By contrast, the theory of social fairness holds that access to needed health care services is a social and community good that should be assured by having each person pay into it regardless of health condition or risk. It rests on a liberal philosophy of justice (Rawls, 1982; Daniels, 1985). The culture and ethics of social fairness seem almost intuitive, rooted in custom and worldview, but a number of manifestations have appeared. Some arguments for social fairness base it on health care as a vital service that restores people (as much as possible) to normal functioning and to the opportunities of life. Other arguments focus on the shared belief that the ill and suffering should always have access to needed services. Some systems based on social fairness charge a flat premium (the most regressive), some a flat wage tax (less regressive), and some an income tax (modestly progressive); but all believe that the healthy should subsidise the ill and the young the old, just as they will be subsidised when they become ill or older.

The BUPA policies threatened to segment the market and force the nation's traditional community-rated insurer either to abandon community rating as well or go bankrupt. For as risk-rated policies draw away healthier subscribers from a community-rated pool, (where the premiums are the same regardless of illnesses, risks, sex or age), the risks and expenses of that pool rise. It must then raise its premiums, which then widens the premium gap and drives still more of the lower risk subscribers to leave. This further exacerbates the problem and by degrees breaks up the community rating pool into pools by risk. The Irish tradition of not discriminating by age or health risk would come to an end, and a spiral of increasing discrimination by risk would begin, as happened in the US market after the Second World War when commercial insurers started risk-rating the traditional community-rated Blue Cross plans, forcing them by turns to behave more and more like risk-rated commercial insurers (Starr, 1982; Light, 1992).

---

1   In the case of driver's insurance, one has only to deal with a few variables and clearer patterns of liability, while in sickness insurance, the interacting risk factors get complex and the resulting expenses less predictable. Also, nearly everyone can drive safely if they want to, while most people do not cause most of their own illnesses.

The campaign

In response to the initial marketing blitz by BUPA to launch its new risk-rated policies, VHI's chairman, Noel Hanlon (1996), wrote to the Minister for Health, Michael Noonan, arguing that the BUPA policies were 'a deliberate attempt to undermine and circumvent the objectives of community rating in the Health Insurance Act 1994'. More darkly, he pointed out that higher premiums for older citizens would lead them to drop their private insurance and 'cause large numbers of high risk persons to fall back upon the public system'. It was urgent, he continued, that the Department determine whether the BUPA cash plans would be allowed to prevail, for they would have 'serious consequences for both VHI and the overall Irish Health Care System'.

In various documented remarks, the Minister, Michael Noonan, said he would defend community rating and review the BUPA policies, but he also said that he welcomed competition 'which has the potential to benefit our market greatly' (Currie, 1996). As is often the case, what kinds of benefits, by what means, were not articulated. Nevertheless, Hanlon had warned against two basic dangers. The new policies would violate the law and values of community rating, and the Department's support of them would ironically force the government to raise taxes to pay for medical services for the older and sicker subscribers who dropped their current policies.

Three weeks later, the *Sunday Business Post* published an excerpt from my speech (Light, 1996) about competition in American health insurance delivered in Dublin the previous October to AIM, an international association of health insurers in 30 nations dedicated to community rating and solidarity (AIM, 1994). The *Post* titled the excerpt 'An unhealthy tale of immorality'. It described how risk-rated policies had drawn off younger groups and eroded the community-rated base of Blue Cross plans until they were forced to risk- and experience-rate themselves. The following Tuesday the Minister for Health reiterated his support of community rating and soon after issued a letter of concern to BUPA. Legislators became increasingly restive, but the Minister continued to fence-sit, saying he would 'decide what further action, if any, is warranted in this matter when BUPA responds to this communication' (Chun an Aire Sláinte, 1996).

Meanwhile, VHI devised a multi-pronged plan to stop BUPA from selling its risk-rated products. It hired a reputable lobbyist and began an intensive legal analysis of the BUPA policies. It began to discuss legislation that would tighten up gaps in the existing law. It hired a consulting firm in public relations and developed several themes: that competition is fine so long as it benefits the Irish people and is fair, but that the BUPA policies harm VHI and the national health system, and undermine family values and solidarity.

Vague and dangerous language was found in BUPA's policies. For example, pre-existing conditions were excluded from reimbursement for medical care and were defined as 'any disease, illness or injury which began before the person . . . started . . . membership' (BUPA Ireland, 1996). This could be interpreted to mean that if a patient were diagnosed with diabetes or cancer after subscribing, but the disease began beforehand, BUPA executives could deny coverage or reimbursement for all medical treatment. Further on, BUPA's rules stated that it would pay benefits only in relation to diagnoses and treatments accepted by medical standards 'as well as to all the circumstances relevant to the person'. Such a vague proviso could allow the insurer not to reimburse medical treat-ment for a wide variety of reasons, including the patient's lifestyle or personal behaviour. The rules also stated that BUPA would not pay for 'treatment, the main purpose or effect of which is to relieve symptoms commonly associated with any bodily change arising from . . . causes such as ageing, menopause or puberty and which is not due to any underlying disease, illness or injury'. This sweeping exclusion could be invoked to exclude from payment medical services for a wide range of serious and costly medical problems of women and of older policyholders.

Four weeks into the campaign, on the eve of Christmas, the Minister finally announced that BUPA's schemes 'may present difficulties as regards the principle of community rating' and that the cash plans are part of 'an integrated insurance package' that may contravene the Health Insurance Act of 1994 (Department of Health, 1996). The phrase, 'integrated insurance package' indicated that the Minister was rejecting BUPA's key argument that its policies consisted of two parts: a community-rated basic insurance part and a risk-rated cash plan. In a separate action, the Attorney General informed the Minister that the policies 'were in breach of community rating legislation' (Wall and Murphy, 1996). BUPA's strategy to define the age-rated cash plans as not insurance and thus outside the level playing field created by the Health Insurance Act had suffered a setback; but its managing director insisted that BUPA's policies were not illegal and said he 'was absolutely confident of the total legality of the organisation's position'.

VHI's chairman warned that if younger people switched to BUPA's cheaper policies, premiums for those over 50 could treble in five years. 'That's what happened in the United States', he added, alluding to the 8 December excerpt of my speech in the *Sunday Business Post. The Times* wrote that BUPA 'is dis-criminating against the elderly and forcing American-style health insurance on Ireland' (Magee, 1996). As is often the case in Europe, American health insurance and the American health care system served as an example of how much more costly and inequitable health care can be.

Despite the Minister's announcement, nothing formally changed. BUPA's risk-rated policies were registered and ready for sale on 1 January 1997. Despite personal inconveniences to the organisers, the campaign's momentum continued through the hallowed Christmas season. The former Taoiseach, Garret FitzGerald

(1996), was moved to publish a prominent essay on 28 December as people talked with each other during the Christmas holidays. He wrote that the BUPA cash plans were a 'very thinly disguised' way to 'evade' the community rating safeguards that would prove 'disastrous' for VHI, since three quarters of its members were under 50, and 'fatal for our health service'.

Nevertheless, sales of the divisive risk-rated policies began right on schedule on 1 January. The Consumers Association of Ireland and the Irish Patients Association believed the policies threatened the interests of sick patients and thought the Minister was failing to uphold societal interests. They therefore attacked the Minister for in effect being the sole stockholder of VHI as well as the regulator of the market, and they called for him to relinquish his role as regulator so that an independent regulator could defend community rating (McNally, 1997). That is, even if the Minister believed that competition was good for VHI, he should not sacrifice community values and solidarity to do so. This battle over moral order and what values should frame health insurance left the thousands of consumers who were interested in BUPA policies in a no man's land, 'a far cry from the government's idea of rejuvenating the Irish health insurance market through competition' (Seekamp and Harding, 1997).

Senior government officials expressed embarrassment at the Minister's slow response and indecision, and the opposition spokeswoman on health for the Dáil said the Minister had handled the affair 'disgracefully'. Then, the *Sunday Business Post* discovered that BUPA had chosen not to submit its policies for prior review before its high-profile launch in November (Seekamp, 1997), suggesting that BUPA had decided to use a blitzkrieg strategy to blast past objections and get its policies on the market, because once in place they would be very hard to remove.

On the morning of 9 January, the seventh week of the campaign, *The Irish Times* published my analysis, as an American expert, that concluded, 'If you believe in fair competition that rewards better value rather than cherry-picking, you need to stop all forms of risk rating before they begin' (Light, 1997a). The analysis described the many direct and indirect ways that risk rating can be done and averred that 'American insurers could drive a herd of Texas long-horns through the vague phrases of the 1994 Act'. This image echoed the Irish saying that one can 'drive a coach-and-four' through an act of parliament, and later that day journalists amused themselves by asking the Irish Minister questions about driving Texas long-horns through the Act. This seemed to butt the Minister off his fence, and that evening he issued a strict warning that BUPA could not issue 'packages' that discriminated against the elderly or ill, and that if it did, it could lead to BUPA losing its licence to trade (Nolan, 1997). Of course, their policies were already being sold. A week later, the Minister announced an 'agreement' with BUPA that it would withdraw its age-rated policies. He also established an independent review body to review any flaws in the community-rated structure of the market (Department of Health, 1997c). The campaign to stop the segmentation of community-based health insurance by risk-rating insurers had succeeded, a rare event in the history of the industry.

Economic and institutional analysis

The Insurance Act of 1994 did more than attempt to foster competition while preserving the cultural repertoire of Irish health insurance. It altered VHI's institutional relationship with the Department of Health fundamentally. As indicated by its origins, the VHI had long been regarded as an extension of the Department, 'an arm of government social policy', as a previous secretary of the Department of Health had put it (Cooper and Smythe, 1997). VHI's services and costs remain highly dependent on the Department, because the government's decisions about how many specialists and surgeons to train, how much to pay them and other staff, what criteria to use for admissions and discharge, and what services to provide all affect the payments that VHI makes. Complicating this dependency, the 1994 Act embodies a paradigm shift to making VHI one in a field of independent competitors. This puts it in an untenable institutional position. If it retains its interdependence with the Department, it either has advantages that make real competition impossible for any outside company, or it is fettered and cannot compete effectively. The Department and government seem deeply ambivalent: they want competition, but not in any form that might threaten the symbolic or financial interdependence between the national health service and VHI.

Cultural ambivalence characterises the European Union as well. Since its directive is silent about community rating or creating a level playing field, is it possible that its authors find discrimination by age and risk acceptable? Do they wish countries to violate the fourth of ten 'benchmarks of fairness' that characterise a health insurance system in a just society (Daniels et al., 1996)? It holds that comprehensive and uniform benefits should be community-rated. This question needs serious and public debate, which constitutes the eighth criterion or benchmark for a fair system. Given how difficult it is to create a level playing field in health insurance, and how modest the administrative overheads are of large insurance systems like the VHI, one wonders if the European Union is barking up the wrong tree with its directive to compete in health insurance. For the major expenses and potential for lowering costs lie in how services are *provided*, and provider competition may be what they are after, though policy makers need to consider evidence from several countries that provider competition increases costs and inequities (Hsiao, 1994; Light, 1997b). In Singapore, Hsiao reports that market competition has led to widespread duplication of expensive medical equipment and high technology services, rapidly rising physician income, and accelerating health care costs. In South Korea, strong demand-side techniques to control rising costs resulted in rapid expansion of unregulated private care which drove up costs at a compound rate in real terms of over 15 per cent per annum. In Chile, market forces introduced to enhance efficiency and contain costs led to (a) a large private market that selects healthy risks and the well-paid workers, (b) a deprivation of the national public system, and (c) worse care for the seriously ill. The Philippines required employers to offer HMOs[2] and offered loans to help HMOs develop, so that they would reduce illness through prevention and hold down the use and costs of hospital and specialty care. Most of the HMOs that developed were for profit, and after a decade the Filipinos found that they charged higher premiums than old-fashioned cost-reimbursement insurance plans, selected the healthy workers and subscribers, and spent only 55 per cent on average on clinical services, using the rest for sales commissions, managers, executive compensation and profits. In the United Kingdom, the welfare structure of the National Health Service (NHS) was transformed into an internal market of competitive contracts following the American model of managed competition. Dangers of bankruptcies and inequalities led the government to limit open competition quickly. Transaction costs rose sharply, and the number of managers tripled. Colleagues became competitors; morale declined. Within a few years, upper-level managers concluded that competition was keeping them from working together to provide good care at low cost, and the competition strategy was largely dropped in favour of managed co-operation (Light, 1997b). In a word, health care does not meet many of the requirements for neoclassical competition so that high transaction costs, fragmentation, privatisation, profiteering and discrimination are likely results (Light, 1995, 1999; Rice, 1998).

The rising premiums of VHI, for example, are not due to its being inefficient, and in fact competition will raise its overhead costs. Thus, the call for competition on the insurance side is based on an inaccurate analysis of why premiums were rising. Rather, VHI's cost problems stem from the high degree to which the medical profession dominates terms of work and payment, and from VHI being piggy-backed on the organisation, culture, financing, and structure of the public system which is strongly centred on hospital-based, specialised services. For example, the Department of Health added considerably more consultants (senior sub-specialists) to the system and increased hospital charges, forcing VHI's costs to rise still faster than they otherwise would

---

2   HMOs stands for health maintenance organisations. These organisations provide, directly or through contracts, all services for their subscribers for a fixed sum per annum per person. This gives them the incentives to prevent as much illness and disability as possible, to teach people how to take care of their own health problems, and to hold down costs.

have (Cooper and Smyth, 1997). VHI is then placed in a no-win position between the resulting cost spiral and minimising premium increases to keep down unrest among its subscribers. As a result, its operating losses exceeded projections for several years during the 1990s, eating up an earlier reserve fund and coming precariously close to not meeting its solvency requirements in what has been characterised as a 'financial meltdown' (n.a. 1997). Yet keeping premiums below the costs of medical services won no friends among subscribers either. They still complained about below-cost increases. Moreover, as a supplementary upgrade that pays significantly more to doctors, VHI policies exacerbate this situation with strong incentives for doctors to hospitalise patients more and do more tests and procedures. Doctors and hospitals check to see if patients have a private insurance card and then increase tests, procedures and fees if they do. In short, substantial solutions to VHI's underlying problems of rising costs and over-utilisation of hospital-based services will require a firm effort to restructure doctor and hospitals payments and jointly developed efforts with the Department to restructure the entire Irish health care system.

The Irish people and their elected officials have shown moral and policy leadership in attempting to ensure that competition in health insurance rewards greater efficiency rather than discrimination against older and sicker citizens. But the law and regulations still leave room for competitors to discriminate even while appearing to community rate. Beyond that, the whole community-rated system, and the social justice it embodies, may be difficult to sustain without strategic adjustments that reward the young for signing up and staying in, and 'punish' older people for not signing up until they are 50 or 55. There are several equitable techniques for dampening these effects, such as age-of-entry community rates and lifetime community rates. Indeed, the reports of the ministerial review recommended changes along these lines (Advisory Group, 1998; Department of Health and Children, 1998).

This has been a study of morals and markets that complements Zelizer's (1985) landmark study in which insurance entrepreneurs created risk-rated markets and priced life, death and the 'priceless child'. Here, moral entrepreneurs and a sociologist intervened against new health insurance policies based on actuarial fairness, highlighted the moral and practical consequences for society, and persuaded the press and politicians to affirm the society's commitment to community-based health insurance. Although we commonly think that money is money, a Euro is a Euro, Zelizer (1994) has shown that we construct many different kinds of money and attribute many different meanings to it. This case concerns how the Dáil attempted to articulate the traditional meaning of health insurance money in the new context of competitive markets, how a new competitor challenged that meaning and began to unravel its institutional manifestation, how a counter offence was mounted, and how the traditional cultural meaning and institutions were reaffirmed, yet permanently altered. *Caveat emptor* was rejected for *confidat emptor*. But the story will continue as the Irish firm up the institutional framework for competition between community-rated insurance policies. This achievement alone makes Ireland a leader among nations that have health insurance markets. If all goes well, it will foster beneficial innovation, improved services, and better controls on costs, while avoiding the hazards of discrimination, dumping and disruption.

Chapter 5

Inequalities in health and health care

Desmond McCluskey

Over several decades, there have been significant improvements in the general health of populations throughout the developed world. Life expectancy – the average number of years to be expected at birth – has increased dramatically. Ireland, too, has shared in this success with a substantial increase in life expectancy and a marked decline in premature deaths (Department of Health and Children, 2003a). However, as in other developed countries, health inequalities between different sections of the population exist in Ireland. The present chapter addresses one such inequality: it focuses specifically on the influence of social class on health and health care.

Social class and health

William Cockerham (1998) cites numerous studies conducted in several European countries as well as in the United States and Canada that point to the marked inequalities in health between different socio-economic groups. In general, people from manual working class backgrounds have higher mortality rates and experience more illness than those from non-manual backgrounds. Disparities are particularly pronounced when one compares the mortality and morbidity rates of the professional and managerial classes with those of the semi-skilled and unskilled groupings. In Britain, the Black Report (Department of Health and Social Security, 1980; Townsend and Davidson, 1982, 1992) indicated that the death rate for adult male unskilled workers was nearly twice that of adult male professional workers. Whitehead (1988, 1992) comments that while death rates in Britain have been declining, rates of chronic illness seem to have been increasing, and the gap in illness rates between manual and non-manual groups has been widening as well, particularly in the over-65 age group. A very good discussion of selected literature relating to the issue of socio-economic status and health chances has been provided by Moore and Harrisson (1995).

Studies of social class and health in Ireland demonstrate a clear relationship between mortality and morbidity rates and social class, as measured by occupational status. A study by Nolan (1990) involved an analysis of mortality rates by socio-economic group for Irish men aged 15 to 64 and was based on Irish Census data for 1981. The results showed significant differentials in standardised mortality rates between men in professional/managerial groups and those in semi-skilled or unskilled occupations – for example, the rate was almost three times as great for unskilled manual workers as for those in the higher professional group – 163 as against 55. Again, from a study by the Institute of Public Health in Ireland, it emerged that there were clear occupational class gradients in all causes of mortality in both the Republic of Ireland and Northern Ireland during the period 1989 to 1998 (Balanda and Wilde, 2001). In both jurisdictions, the annual directly standardised mortality rate in the lowest occupational class was significantly higher (over 130 per cent) than the rate in the highest occupational class.

A second study by Nolan focused on morbidity rates (Nolan, 1991). It was based on data obtained in a large-scale national household survey carried out by the Economic and Social Research Institute (ESRI) in 1987. The data covered the presence or absence of major chronic illness or infirmity, as reported by the respondents. Sharp differentials across the social classes in the percentages reporting chronic illness were found: as in other countries, those from semi-skilled and unskilled manual social classes were considerably more likely than others to have experienced major illness or infirmity. The percentage of respondents reporting such illness in the various age groups was at least twice as high for the unskilled manual as for the professional and managerial class. A similar picture emerged from a study by McCluskey (1989): reports of major illness were associated more with respondents from manual than from non-manual occupations and more common among those with lower levels of educational attainment than among those with higher levels.

Studies of the relationship between social class and health status in Ireland are quite limited in number. However, some few other studies that have been carried out are listed by the Public Health Alliance of Ireland (PHAI) (Burke et al., 2004), and include the following: Travellers, a group that has traditionally led a nomadic lifestyle,[1] live on average 11 years less than settled people (Barry, 1989); children from lower income groups are most likely to have accidents in the home (Laffoy, 1997); in 1999 the perinatal mortality rate was three times higher for children of unskilled manual workers than for those born in the higher professional category (Cullen, 2002); in 1996, men in unskilled jobs were eight times more likely to die from an accidental cause than men in the higher professions (Barry et al., 2001); men in unskilled jobs were four times more likely to be admitted to hospital for schizophrenia than higher professional workers (Barry et al., 2001).

1   Travellers form a community whose members traditionally have led a nomadic lifestyle, travelling in caravans or mobile homes. Many now live in settled accommodation.

The Black Report (Department of Health and Social Security, 1980) and The Health Divide (Whitehead, 1988) refer to four types of explanation of social class differences in health.

The *artefact explanation* suggests that both health and class are artefact variables thrown up by attempts to measure social phenomena, and that the relationship between them may be an artefact of little causal significance. As Gillespie and Prior (1995: 202) summarise the argument: 'any apparent "cause and effect" relation between social class and health is dismissed as a measurement artefact – produced by indifferent health and mortality data and an inadequate/ inconsistent classification of social classes.' However, these same writers comment that since so much research by different parties, using different methods at different times, has found a consistent association between 'class' (however defined) and health, it seems illogical to dismiss this as an aberration of figures. In other words, very real differences in health exist between social groups which cannot be explained away as an artefact.

Theories of *natural and social selection* suggest that people in poor health tend to drift down the occupational scale and concentrate in the lower social strata while people in good health tend to move up into higher classes. Health problems therefore precede social location, rather than flow from it. And, as Gillespie and Prior (1995: 202) observe, 'Since some causes of ill health are genetically transmitted, this social selection will be reinforced by *natural* selection, as a predisposition to ill/good health is passed on from one generation to the next.' They point out, however, that the major difficulty with the selection argument is the lack of evidence to support it. As David Blane summarises the position: 'the contribution of health-related social mobility to social class differences in health is probably small' (Blane, 1997: 117).

The *cultural/behavioural* explanation suggests that inherent in working-class culture are patterns of behaviour detrimental to health. More specifically, people of lower socio-economic status are more likely than those of higher levels to damage their health by the consumption of refined food, tobacco and alcohol, by lack of exercise and by the underutilisation of preventive health care. Black (Department of Health and Social Security, 1980) and Whitehead (1988) accept that variations in lifestyle could indeed account for some of the class differential in health. Notable examples would be the greater prevalence of cigarette smoking and the lower uptake of preventive services among those from manual working-class backgrounds, which could translate into poorer health. However, Black and Whitehead concur that behavioural differences could by no means account for all of the health differential between social classes. As Whitehead records, when studies are able to control for factors like smoking and drinking, a sizeable gap remains. She notes, indeed, that in some cases *most* of the difference in health is not explained by lifestyle factors.

The *structuralist/materialist* explanation proposes that health inequalities can best be understood in terms of the material consequences of the class structure. In general, people in lower socio-economic groups are exposed to a more unhealthy environment: they do more dangerous work, are more susceptible to unemployment, have poorer housing, and have fewer resources available to secure the necessities for health. While accepting that the very poor, those who are extremely deprived, would be most at risk, the emphasis is largely on *relative* disadvantage. Though people today in lower occupational groups, with lower incomes, are likely to be experiencing better health than their counterparts of past generations, at the same time they are likely to be disadvantaged in terms of health when compared with their contemporaries in higher occupational groups, on higher levels of income.

The Black Report (Department of Health and Social Security, 1980), having reviewed the evidence for the various explanations, concludes that health inequalities are explained more by structuralist/ materialist factors than by any other. Nolan (1994) and Whitehead (1988) take a similar view, pointing to the growing body of evidence which indicates that material and structural factors such as housing and income can have a marked impact on health. 'Most importantly', Whitehead argues, 'several studies have shown how adverse social conditions can limit the choice of lifestyle and it is this set of studies which illustrates most clearly that behaviour cannot be separated from its social context. Certain living and working conditions appear to impose severe restrictions on an individual's ability to choose a healthy lifestyle' (Whitehead, 1988: 336). Explanations of health inequalities which concentrate on behaviour considered health-damaging may fail to recognise the adverse social conditions from which such behaviour may have arisen. For example, Whitehead points to studies that have found lack of money to be a major factor restricting food choice, as well as the quantity of food consumed. She also cites research findings which highlighted the use of smoking by women to help them survive their stressful workload. Gillespie and Prior summarise the argument most succinctly: 'Those on very low incomes may have far less choice about where and how they live' (Gillespie and Prior, 1995: 203). And as Jones (1994) warns, targeting individual lifestyle can come close to 'blaming the victims', if people are in a position where change is very difficult or even impossible.

Whitehead (1988) stresses that the two approaches, the lifestyle and the material, are interrelated rather than mutually exclusive. An emphasis, therefore, on the relationship between behavioural and material factors may be perceived as the way forward for reducing health inequalities. However, Davey Smith et al. (1990) reject this approach, since it tends to discount any influence of the social and material environment that is not mediated through behavioural patterns; intervention is seen largely in terms of encouraging changes in lifestyle, thus distracting attention away from the necessity of effecting change

in the environment. Others, more recently, have expressed considerable opposition to any such polarisation of views. Popay and her associates (Popay et al.,
1998), while they are critical of studies which disconnect individuals from their
social context, at the same time emphasise the importance of focusing on
individual lived experience. They call attention to the proposal of Macintyre
(1997) that studies of health inequalities require a move to a more micro-level
examination of the pathways by which social structure influences mental and
physical health. Such an approach would counteract the determinism inherent
in structuralist analyses where, according to Kelly and Charlton (1995), 'the
individual is relegated to being nothing more than a system outcome, not a
thinking human being' (1995: 83). The foregoing controversy reflects the classic
sociological problem of structure and agency.

Social class and health care

The complex nature of the explanation of health inequalities is further
demonstrated when one considers the question of access to and use of health
services. International evidence points to lower socio-economic groups being
less likely than others to make use of preventive care (see chapter 14). On the
other hand, where the focus is on *illness* behaviour, many studies in the United
States and Britain, indicate that, when ill, people in lower income groups
and in lower occupational classes are higher utilisers of medical services (see
Cockerham, 1998; Whitehead, 1988). This is particularly true of General
Practitioner (GP) consultations but the evidence also suggests greater use of
both outpatient and inpatient hospital services by the manual working class.

However, it is argued that when usage of services is related to actual *need*,
then working-class people use fewer services relative to their needs. In the
United States, where in 1995 approximately 40 million people lacked health
insurance coverage, access to quality medical care is still a problem for a number of disadvantaged groups (Cockerham, 1998). Whitehead (1988) observes
that in the United Kingdom, where there is universal entitlement to the
National Health Service, this does not always guarantee access to such services
in practice. There is evidence to support the claim of Tudor Hart (1971) that an
inverse care law applies, that the provision of health care is inversely related to
the need for it: those areas with greatest health need have the poorest provision
of services. Moreover, Whitehead (1992) notes that there is also evidence to
indicate that people from working-class backgrounds experience an inferior
quality of service. Studies have shown that patients in higher socio-economic
groups received more explanations voluntarily from their GPs, more frequently
had home visits, and were more likely to have been referred to specialist services.
'This', Whitehead suggests, 'leads to the more general question about whether

higher social classes receive more effective treatment and whether that is a contributing factor in the differential in survival chances of people from different social classes' (Whitehead, 1992: 280).

Irish studies by Tussing (1985), McCluskey (1989) and Nolan (1991) showed higher GP consulting rates for those on lower incomes. But again, there is the question of whether this uptake, especially by the poor, matches their greater need. Nolan's analysis (1991) showed that even when one controlled for their higher incidence of ill-health, those from lower income groups were more likely than others to have consulted a doctor within a specific twelve-month period and to have done so on more occasions within that time space. However, as the author concedes, this finding could be due partly to the fact that the measures of ill health employed were crude and underestimated the incidence of illness among lower income groups.

Health care in Ireland is a mix of public and private provision. As Nolan (1991) observes, the relationship is not one between two parallel systems; rather, the private and public elements are intertwined. At present, there are two categories of eligibility for public services. People in Category I, the lower income group accounting for somewhat less than one third of the population, are issued with medical cards which entitle them and their dependants to all services free of charge.[2] Those in Category II, the rest of the population, are entitled to a free hospital service in public wards of publicly funded hospitals, but do not qualify for free general practitioner services as do those in Category I. Despite the fact that the entire population is entitled to free hospital care, 46 per cent of the population were covered by private health insurance in 2001. This provides patients with private or semi-private hospital accommodation and choice of consultant. But, according to the Report of the Commission on Health Funding (1989), the main reasons why people take up private medical insurance is the perception that private care, whether in a public or private hospital, carries with it faster access to treatment and higher quality care – the latter being represented by a greater degree of personal attention from the consultant rather than from junior medical staff. The findings of an ESRI study (Nolan and Wiley, 2000) present a similar picture. About 43 per cent of 2,620 people surveyed reported that they had taken out private health insurance. Of these, over three quarters indicated that they had done so to gain faster access to hospital services when needed, and one in five to be sure of getting good quality treatment. The authors of the Report of the Commission on Health Funding stated that they were in no doubt that the public perception was an accurate one, and that in some cases, speedy access to necessary treatment was determined by the ability to pay, rather than by medical need. This issue was highlighted at a conference on Health Inequalities and Poverty organised by the Society of St Vincent De

2   In 2001, eligibility for medical cards was extended to all aged over 70, regardless of income.

Paul (SVP) in 2000. A report of the conference in *The Irish Times* (Ó Moráin, 2000a) describes vividly experiences of public patients when confronted with obstacles to treatment. In one instance, a woman with gangrene in both feet was told she would have to wait five weeks for a hospital bed – but when the SVP offered to pay for her accommodation, a bed was found immediately. Another case, cited in the *Opinion* section of the same newspaper (Ó Moráin, 2000b), was that of a young boy, four years of age, who had to wait for a year for an appointment with an ear specialist. While waiting, his preventable condition worsened to the point where he developed a speech problem. He was then placed on a waiting list for speech therapy. The author of the newspaper report cynically commented, 'When the health system says we don't have the capacity to treat you for six weeks or six months or two years, is it really saying something like: "We have the capacity to treat you straight away but we are keeping it to one side for people who can pay. If you can't pay, tough"' (Ó Moráin, 2000b: 14). To remove inequalities of access to hospital treatment, the Commission on Health Funding in 1989 urged the adoption of common waiting lists for public and private patients, but this recommendation has not been implemented.

In November 2001, in the face of mounting criticism of the health system, the Irish government launched a National Health Strategy, having among its principal aims the provision of a fully integrated primary care service and the cutting of hospital waiting lists. In the introduction to the document, it was admitted that very clear deficiencies in services existed, including unacceptably long waiting times in various parts of the system.

The National Health Strategy 2001

'The new National Health Strategy, *Quality and Fairness: A Health System for You*, outlines the largest concentrated expansion in services in the history of the Irish health system' (Department of Health and Children, 2001a: 11). The costings of the programme were estimated at just over €12.7 billion, as expressed in 2001 prices.

The Strategy set out four national goals to guide activity and planning in the health system, for the years 2002 to 2011: better health for everyone; fair access; responsive and appropriate care delivery; high performance. In respect of fair access, the Strategy stated: 'Fair access is concerned with ensuring that equal access for equal need is a core value for the delivery of public funded services' (2001a: 74). All patients should have access to a high quality service within a reasonable period of time irrespective of whether they were public or private patients.

To achieve the four national goals, a series of essential actions were identified under six frameworks for change, including strengthening primary care and reform of the acute hospital system. Since much of the controversy concerning health inequalities in the utilisation of services relates to access to hospital care, the discussion which follows will focus largely on the proposed reform of the hospital system. (For proposed changes for strengthening primary care, see Curry, chapter 1.)

Reform of the acute hospital system

At the outset, it is observed that the number of acute hospital inpatient beds in Ireland has decreased from 17,665 in 1980, to 11,862 in the year 2000. Despite this, activity levels were increased by steps such as reducing average lengths of stay, a huge increase in day activities, and making use of new technology. However, increases in the total population, including a rise in the number of older people and overall growth in demand for services, point to a need for additional capacity and, more specifically, an expansion in bed numbers. The Strategy document stated that it was clear that waiting times for some elective (non-emergency) treatments were unacceptably long. In this respect, glaring inequalities are found between public and private patients. The document noted that the position of public patients in public hospitals relative to private patients had deteriorated in recent years. The Strategy addressed these problems under three headings: capacity, efficiency, and equity.

Capacity

Over the ten-year period to the end of 2011, a total of 3,000 acute beds will be added to the hospital system. As many as 650 extra beds were to be provided by the end of 2002, with 450 in the public sector. At the same time, the private sector would be contracted to provide a further 200 beds, all for the treatment of public patients on waiting lists.

To help determine the specialities in which these extra beds would be provided and their location around the country a National Hospitals Agency would be established on a statutory footing. The Agency would advise the Minister and the Department of Health and Children on the general organisation, planning and co-ordination of acute hospital services. It would also develop a national waiting time database to help channel patients awaiting treatment to an appropriate hospital with sufficient capacity. An important part of the Agency's role, in collaboration with the health boards and the Eastern Regional Health Authority, would be to promote closer working relationships between the public and private hospital sectors.

Efficiency

The Strategy set out a comprehensive series of actions to be taken to reduce waiting times for public patients. Among the specified targets, it was stated: 'By the end of 2004, no public patients would wait longer than three months for treatment following referral from an out-patient department.' This target was to be achieved largely by the major expansion in acute bed capacity, referred to above. Two other actions, a new ear-marked Treatment Purchase Fund and substantial improvements in Accident and Emergency (A&E) services, were also designed to make a significant contribution to the reduction in waiting times.

The Treatment Purchase Fund would be used to purchase treatment from private hospitals in Ireland and from international providers specifically for public patients who have waited more than three months from their outpatient appointment. The Fund would be managed by a National Treatment Purchase Team appointed by the Minister for Health and Children. It would work in partnership with the health boards, hospitals, and consultants to ensure that waiting times for public patients are reduced as quickly as possible. Where it is not possible to treat patients within a reasonable period in Ireland, either in public or private hospitals, arrangements will be made to refer public patients for treatment abroad, taking into account quality, availability and cost.

Major improvements in Accident and Emergency departments are also perceived as playing an important part in reducing waiting lists. Additional A&E consultants will be appointed to organise and run A&E departments. This will expedite clinical decision making and enhance diagnosis and treatment. Triage procedures – initial rapid assessments – will help prioritise patients according to their needs and channel them quickly to the most appropriate form of care.

The National Hospitals Agency is to play a major role, as well, in reform of the management and organisation of waiting lists. Working with the health boards and the ERHA, and in consultation with professional bodies, it will lead the development of guidelines for referral and prioritisation of patients within and between specialities.

Equity
The Strategy stressed that both public and private patients were entitled to care within a reasonable period of time. The challenge, therefore, is to ensure that a fair balance is achieved and that those dependent on the public system are not disadvantaged. As well as the measures referred to above under the headings of *capacity* and *efficiency* and identified as promoting *equity*, additional actions are specified to address this issue and the mix between public and private care. In this connection, the Strategy drew attention to the contractual right of hospital consultants to carry out private practice in public hospitals. It identified the terms of the common contract as central to the establishment of an appropriate balance between public and private hospital care. Therefore, negotiations on changes to the contract had to involve restructuring key elements of the current system, including more flexible work practices, to provide equity of access. One proposed measure was that newly appointed consultants work exclusively for public patients for a specified number of years.

As a further step to improve equity for public patients, the health boards and the ERHA were to monitor hospital performance on waiting times. If these bodies concluded that targets for reduction of waiting times were not being achieved, a hospital would be directed to suspend admission of private patients for elective procedures in a speciality until the waiting time for public patients was restored to within the target period of time. However, this direction could be set aside if hospital management and the consultants could agree on alternative means of restoring the target waiting time. This was seen as an important measure since it provided an incentive for hospitals and consultants to use all available means to address unacceptably long waiting times.

Another measure mooted in the Strategy to promote fair access to health services was the proposal to increase significantly the number of people covered by the medical card scheme. At the launch of the Strategy, the then Minister for Health and Children, Micheál Martin, stated that it was his intention to extend medical card eligibility to 200,000 extra people in 2003. This promise did not progress until 2004 (see Curry, chapter 1 above).

Finally, in the Health Strategy document, there was a commitment to implement a series of actions to achieve the National Anti-Poverty Strategy (1997) health programme, that is, to eliminate the impact of deprivation and disadvantage on health status. Four targets were set out: (i) the gap in premature mortality between the lowest and highest socio-economic groups to be reduced by at least 10 per cent for circulatory diseases, cancers, injuries and poisoning by 2007; (ii) the gap in life expectancy between Travellers and the whole population to be reduced by at least 10 per cent by 2007; (iii) the life expectancy and health status of Travellers to be monitored so that by 2003, existing targets can be reviewed and revised; (iv) by 2007, the gap in low birth weight rates between children from the lowest and highest socio-economic groups to be reduced by 10 per cent from the current level.

Reaction to the Health Strategy

On its publication, the Health Strategy was, initially, generally welcomed by the media, by most health-care professional bodies and by consumer organisations (although with reservations, indeed major reservations, by some commentators). These various groups were wholehearted in their support for the new model of primary care (see Department of Health and Children, 2001b). However, the Strategy's programme for the reform of the acute hospital system generated considerable criticism because it is in this area that inequalities in the health services are most clearly seen. For this reason the critique which follows focuses primarily on this element of the Strategy.

One of the most important analyses of the Strategy document was that of the National Economic and Social Forum (NESF) in its report, *Equity of Access to Hospital Care* (NESF, 2002). Though broadly welcoming the Strategy, the report voiced a number of concerns relating to its implementation, prompting NESF to make the following recommendations: that waiting-list targets should not be met through 'wait shifting' (that is, reducing waits between out-patient consultation and treatment by increasing waits between GP referral and out-patient consultation); that it was essential that legislation be enacted to guarantee rights to treatment within a reasonable period, taking into account the limits of the public resources available for the health services; that access to public hospitals should be on the basis of a common waiting list (otherwise the underlying inequality in the system will continue); that common standards should be established and regulated in both the public and private sectors; that alternative models of care in other countries that do not have the same equity problems should be independently investigated.

Critique of the Irish Health System

Subsequent to the NESF report, a most comprehensive critique of the Irish Health System, *Unhealthy State* (2003) by Maev-Ann Wren, was published. Wren observes that the greatest barrier to access to hospital care for people on low incomes is that the hospital system has been so poorly resourced that care is rationed and the rationing is according to income, not need. She points out that while emergency cases are treated on a first-come, first-served basis, all other public hospital care is channelled through two distinct routes: a fast track for private patients who have private insurance, and slow public waiting lists for the rest. Public patients may wait years for treatment which private patients may receive within weeks. Further, when they reach hospital, public patients may also experience inferior treatment. According to Wren, this two-tier system of access and care is rooted in how hospitals are organised and how doctors are employed and work. It reflects 'deliberate government policy, expressed in the system of bed designation and the traditional work practices and self-interest of hospital consultants, expressed in their common contract' (Wren, 2003: 175).

A general assessment of the Health Strategy, 2001

Sociologists of health and medicine should find a great deal to commend in the 2001 Health Strategy document (Department of Health and Children, 2001a). Much of its thinking reflected the sociological approach, and indeed many of the concepts it employed were borrowed from the social sciences, such as empowerment, holism, lifestyles and social capital. Above all, sociologists should welcome its commitment to a health system based on a social rather than on a biomedical model of health. The theme of quality of life informed the entire Strategy document: 'The definition of health used in this Strategy places value on quality of life; the emphasis will not be on medical status alone' (2001a: 16) and 'Addressing quality of life issues must be a central objective of the Health Strategy' (2001a: 61).

Consistent with its emphasis on the social model of health the Strategy stressed that in developing an effective health system account had to be taken of the social, economic, environmental and cultural factors which influence health. It recognised, as has been shown in many sociological and epidemio-logical studies, that people from lower socio-economic groups suffer a disproportionate burden of ill health; that educational, housing and nutritional deprivation affect both an individual's health status and his or her ability to access services. Hence, the Strategy declared: 'Equity will be central to deve-loping policies, (i) to reduce the difference in health status currently running across the social spectrum in Ireland, and (ii) to ensure equitable access to services based on need' (2001a: 18). More specifically, it stressed that tackling health inequalities was inextricably linked with tackling issues of poverty. Moreover, the concern would not only be with addressing the health inequalities of those of lower socio-economic status but also with attending to the needs of particular groups such as the elderly, people with disabilities, members of the Travelling community, people with mental illness and those with chronic conditions. The stated goal was to ensure that everyone in society had an equal chance to achieve his or her full health potential. Sociologists should very much welcome this emphasis on equality since issues of unequal access to health and health care tend to occupy centre-stage in most, if not all, sociological analyses of health policy and health care.

The Strategy's declaration that a people-centred approach will be a key principle of the programme is also to be welcomed. A people-centred approach means improving the 'patient focus' so that the health system responds to the needs of consumers, to patients and clients, rather than consumers having to conform to the way the system works. Lack of integration of care between and even within some services is identified in the Strategy as a problem in existing services. It acknowledges that individual patients or clients may have to access the system several times to have all their needs addressed. The Strategy concludes that if the system is to be responsive to the needs of individuals, it is important that a holistic or whole-person approach is taken to planning and delivering care. A holistic approach denotes not only the integration of services in the interest of consumers but also seeing patients and clients in their social and cultural context and giving due attention to their psychological as well as their physical state.

A people-centred approach also implies the empowerment of people to be active participants in decisions relating to their health. In the Health Strategy it is stated at the outset that the vision of the future health system was one that 'encourages you to have your say, listens to you, and ensures that your views are taken into account'. In discussing its third national goal, responsive and appropriate care delivery, it was emphasised that health and social care personnel should encourage shared decision making and, where possible, accommodate patient preferences. Further, there was a commitment to carrying out routine patient satisfaction surveys and to the collection and analysis of complaints so that the results would inform local decision making.

Most of the actions proposed in the Strategy were generally welcomed. At the same time, many have been less than happy with two features of the programme which appear inconsistent with the national goal of fair access, that is, ensuring that equal access for equal need is a core value for the delivery of publicly funded services. In the first place, though the measures to reduce hospital waiting lists were well received, there has been considerable criticism of the policy to retain the 'two-tiered' system of hospital care, which results in private patients having speedier access to elective treatment than public patients. Secondly, there was major disappointment with the decision not to implement immediately, following the Strategy's publication, the plan to substantially increase the number of people covered by the medical card scheme. Further, towards the end of 2002, it was announced that a government promise to extend the medical card scheme to an additional 200,000 people was to be postponed. Eventually, the Minister for Finance, in the Book of Estimates 2004, announced that around 230,000 additional medical cards would be issued. However, about 200,000 of these would entitle their holders to a General Practitioner-only service, but would not include the cost of medicines. The remaining 30,000 would receive the full medical card, which covers free GP visits and medicines. Then, in May 2005, at the Conference of the Irish College of General Practitioners, Mary Harney, appointed Minister for Health and Children in succession to Micheál Martin, announced that the issuing of the extra medical cards would be fast-tracked, and that in future all applicants for medical cards, including the doctor-only cards, would be assessed on the basis of *disposable* income – mortgage or rent costs, transport and childcare costs, would be taken into account.

To the above two criticisms, one might add what could be considered a serious omission from the Strategy. Though the Strategy document noted that, while the Health Act 1970 explicitly provided for eligibility for a service, it did not provide for a person being entitled to receive a service. This means that, currently, there is no statutory framework underpinning access to services within a stated timeframe. It was proposed, therefore, in the Strategy that new legislation would move away from the rather theoretical model of 'eligibility', to a system of entitlement to services within a reasonable period of time. But nowhere in the Strategy document was it stated that health was a fundamental human right, which, of course, would imply full access to quality health services for all, based solely on need.

Changes in the economy

Since its launch at the end of 2001, a temporary reduction in exchequer returns and a decline in economic growth posed a threat to the Strategy's full implementation. This pessimism was fuelled by a number of governmental decisions in the second half of 2002. Among these was the directive to the health boards not to fill 800 newly approved administrative and managerial posts and perhaps, even more significantly, the announcement towards the end of the year, as mentioned above, of the postponement of a Programme for Government promise to extend the medical card scheme in 2003 to an additional 200,000 people on low incomes. Also seen as reflecting the impact of the worsened economic circumstances on health provision were the decisions to raise the threshold of the drug refund scheme and to increase accident and emergency charges. Lack of adequate funding, too, has been identified as a major factor in the deteriorating conditions faced in Accident & Emergency (A&E) departments of hospitals. It is not uncommon in A&E departments for patients, diagnosed as requiring hospitalisation, to spend many hours, even days, on hospital trolleys before being admitted to wards because of delayed discharges. Patients ready for discharge continue to occupy acute beds because necessary step-down facilities – convalescent services in nursing homes or in the community – have not been provided by health boards, allegedly, as a result of budgetary constraints.

The strongest criticism both from the media and the political opposition parties has been directed at the failure of the government to meet the targets specified in the Strategy to reduce waiting times for public patients. The government's promise that by the end of 2004 no public patient would wait longer than six months and no child longer than three months for treatment following referral from an outpatient department, was not met.

The Health Service Reform Programme 2003

A significant event occurred in 2003 which, more than anything else, will have major implications for the achievement of the National Health Strategy's goals. On 18 June 2003, the government announced radical reforms in the Irish Health Service. In the Introduction to the proposed reforms, the then Minister for Health and Children, Micheál Martin, emphasised the importance of having 'the right organisational structures and management practices in place so that we can actually achieve the objectives set out in the strategy'. The reforms are based on the findings of two reports: *Commission on Financial Management and Control Systems in the Health Service* (Brennan Report) commissioned by the Department of Finance, and *Audit of Structures and Functions in the Health System* (Prospectus Report). The government plan published under the title *The Health Service Reform Programme* (Department of Health and Children, 2003c) contains a number of key elements (see Curry, chapter 1 above).

Without question, the most radical measure of the programme was the decision to abolish the existing health board/authority structures and to subsume their functions into a new body, the Health Service Executive (HSE) outside the Department of Health and Children – the first ever body charged with managing the health service as a single, national entity. Such a radical restructuring of the system was not intimated in the Health Strategy (2001) and was certainly not part of its immediate agenda.

A third major report relating to the reform of the Irish Health Service, that of the *National Task Force on Medical Staffing* (Hanly Report) (Department of Health and Children, 2003b) was also published in July 2003, but subsequent to the *Health Service Reform Programme*. The Minister, Micheál Martin, declared that its conclusions 'fitted like a glove' into the reforms sought by the Brennan and Prospectus documents. Among its recommendations were that acute hospital services be organised on a regional basis, and that there should be a major increase in the number of hospital consultants to bring about a consultant-provided, rather than a consultant-led, service. This second measure would require a renegotiation of consultants' contracts.

Conclusion

The changes planned in the National Health Strategy 2001 and in the Health Service Reform Programme 2003, together with the proposals of the Hanly Report, represent the biggest overhaul of the health services in 30 years. From statements in the media, it is apparent that the government is going to meet with stubborn opposition from professional, sectional, and local interest groups as it seeks to implement its plans. Whatever the outcome of these struggles, it is clear that the first decade of the new millennium will witness significant changes in the organisation and delivery of health care in Ireland. It would appear equally clear that other radical changes will be required if the glaring inequalities between public and private patients are to be tackled and the core value of the National Health Strategy – of equal access for equal need – is to be realised.

Part 2

The nursing role

Chapter 6

Development of the role of the nurse in Ireland

Gerard M. Fealy

The turn of the twenty-first century was a period of enormous change for the nursing profession in Ireland. In the preceding decade, the profession had undergone a level of development that it had not experienced in its previous one hundred years and the result of this development was that nursing in Ireland had joined the ranks of the graduate professions in health care. How did Irish nursing achieve this position? By exploring the development of modern nursing in Ireland, this chapter attempts to answer this question.

Nursing reform and professional regulation

In the nineteenth century, the voluntary hospitals were the principal means of providing indoor medical relief for the growing populations of urban poor. Through their association with the medical schools of the city, the Dublin voluntary hospitals participated in important advances in hospital scientific medicine (O'Brien, 1984); in a fifty-year period beginning at about 1820, Dublin became a world-renowned centre for medical education, when the so-called Dublin Medical School flourished (McGeachie, 1999).

While the work of the Dublin Medical School led to the development of new methods in the diagnosis and treatment of disease, the nursing care did not keep pace with the advances made in the period; in the voluntary hospitals, women with no formal training in sick nursing provided the nursing care (Fealy, 2002a). Being of the servant class, the behaviour of the nurse was attributed to her class and 'great evils' were associated with the conduct of untrained nurses (House of Commons, 1854); there were reports of sluttish behaviour, drunkenness, inefficient nursing, and neglect of duty (Fealy, 2002a). After about 1880, there began a process of nursing and sanitary reform that would, by the century's end, result in the replacement of the great majority of untrained nurses with a 'better class' of nurse, a lady nurse drawn from the middle and lower middle classes. Hospital probationership training was a key part of this reform process. Initiated by Anglo-Irish Protestant social reformers, the reform of nursing was driven by the need to have a skilled nurse to meet the needs of patients and medical men, arising in the wake of the advances in scientific medicine (Fealy, 2002a).

While the reform of nursing in Ireland had transformed the care of the hospitalised sick, a woman could still present herself for employment as a nurse without having received proper training. The public could not be assured that the nurse was properly trained and there were reports of untrained nurses passing themselves off as 'properly trained' nurses. In an attempt to bring about an end to this situation, a campaign to achieve state regulation of nursing commenced in the late nineteenth century. The campaign sought professional regulation through state registration and the regulation and standardisation of nurse training. The campaign was an international endeavour, involving a range of vested interests including nurses, the medical profession, the voluntary hospitals, the workhouse infirmaries, and private nursing homes (Abel-Smith, 1960). A number of Irish nursing leaders, most notably Margaret Huxley, Matron of Sir Patrick Dun's Hospital, played a prominent role in the so-called 'battle for registration' (McGann, 1992). Huxley argued that a standardised system of nurse training, under the control of a state regulatory authority, would safeguard the public from untrained and unsafe nurses (House of Commons, 1905).

The campaign for state registration was a natural continuation of the process of nursing and sanitary reform, but owing to a number of interrelated factors, including vested self-interests among the voluntary hospitals and the medical profession, professional disunity, and the First World War, the campaign lasted for some thirty years. The campaign finally attained its goal of state regulation of nursing when the Nurses Registration (Ireland) Act was enacted in 1919.

State registration was the final act in the reform of nursing, placing nursing in Ireland on a professional footing. The entry of intelligent and influential women into leadership positions in nursing, the improved quality of care that nursing reform had brought, and the contribution that nurses made to First World War, meant that nursing was held in high public esteem, and this high social standing of the nurse contributed to the eventual attainment of professional regulation (Fealy, 2002a). The campaign for state registration also coincided with the campaign for the movement for women's suffrage (Griffon, 1994), and it was an expression of the 'female professional project' (Witz, 1992).

General Nursing Council for Ireland, 1920–49

Professional regulation was the single most important event in the development of modern nursing in Ireland; the General Nursing Council for Ireland was the new body with responsibility for maintaining a register of nurses and setting down the standards for nurse training and examinations. Established under the Nurses Registration (Ireland) Act, the Council regulated the new nursing profession in Ireland between 1920 and 1950.

Among the principal concerns of the Council were the need to obtain reciprocity with English and other international regulatory authorities, and the need to develop a national standardised system of training. By 1923, the Council had put in place all of the necessary structures for standardised training, including a syllabus of training and regulations as to how hospitals should organise and conduct nurse training (General Nursing Council for Ireland, 1923). While the Council did not have control over the recruitment of nurses, in its early years it was concerned with patronage in the selection of candidates for nursing (Fealy, 2002a). In 1926, the Council expressed disquiet at the 'practice of Boards of Health interfering with the Doctors and Matrons in the selection of Probationer Nurses', resulting in candidates being selected, regardless of their fitness (General Nursing Council, 1926). Thus, while the nursing profession in Ireland now controlled its own affairs in theory, in practice other vested interests were controlling the affairs of nursing. In the areas of recruitment and selection, the organisation of the curriculum of training, and conditions of employment, the nurses' employers were the principal controllers; the voluntary hospitals, in particular, tended to adopt a position of independence vis-à-vis the state and statutory bodies like the General Nursing Council (Daly, 1999). Thus, despite registration legislation, the campaign for professional regulation did not attain the sort of autonomy and control of nursing affairs that the advocates of state registration had envisaged (Witz, 1992).

Nor was the putative new professional status that nurses derived from professional regulation reflected in their economic position; for much of the first thirty years following state registration, nurses in Ireland experienced poor conditions of employment, related principally to the poor economic circumstances that prevailed following Irish independence, but also related to the general undervaluing of the work of caring. The intrinsic satisfaction that nurses derived from their work was seen as sufficient recompense to supplement their paltry salary (O'Sullivan, 1964). The work of nursing in Ireland was linked to women's work and sick nursing exemplified an extension of women's domestic and familial activities related to caring, residing in the realm of gendered, paid employment (O'Connor, 1998). Nursing had a low value in the economy and the intelligence required for much of the work of nursing went unrecognised (O'Connor, 1998). Notwithstanding the considerable economic hardship experienced by nurses in the thirty years after the establishment of the General Nursing Council for Ireland, the voluntary hospitals had no difficulty in recruiting young women into nursing.

Development of nursing after 1950

The Nurses Act 1950 replaced the General Nursing Council for Ireland with a new professional regulatory authority, An Bórd Altranais (The Nursing Board). The Council was replaced at a time when the notion of a welfare state was emerging in Britain and in Ireland (Robins, 2000). Influenced by the Beveridge Report, which was published in the United Kingdom in 1942, Irish government policy in the late 1940s was aimed at providing a universal, publicly funded health service. Nurses and midwives would play their part in the new services and it was envisaged that nurses would become more involved in disease prevention and health education. The purpose of the Nurses Act was therefore to bring nursing and midwifery under a single regulatory authority and to provide for rational recruitment and training of nurses to meet the demands for nursing service in the expanding health services (Deeny, 1949). However, under the new Nursing Board, nurse training failed to reflect the new roles envisioned for nurses; the role of hospital nurse, with its emphasis on nursing in illness, continued to be the focus of the nurse training programme, and recruitment to nursing continued to be undertaken by the hospitals, solely on the basis of their own local service needs (Fealy, 2002a).

The over-emphasis on illness at the expense of health promotion in the training of nurses increasingly became a matter of concern to nursing internationally after 1950. Meeting in Brussels in 1955, a World Health Organisation study group called for a broad-based curriculum that prepared the nurse for her responsibilities not only towards the ill person, but also towards the healthy (Anon., 1955). A related concern in the training of nurses was the impact that the status of the trainee nurse as a hospital employee was having on her learning, and there were calls to separate nurse training and nursing service and to afford student nurses full student status. In Ireland, however, there was a general recognition that Irish hospitals could not function without the services provided by the labour of student nurses (Elms et al., 1974).

Clinical practice

All the while, medical science and the increasing array of medical services being provided in the large acute general hospitals were driving the development and the direction of the Irish health services, and nursing was intimately tied into this project. In the 1960s and 1970s, Irish nurses successfully embraced the new technologies in health care and played an active role in developing their nursing skills to meet the needs of patients undergoing a range of new diagnostic and therapeutic procedures. Recruitment to nursing reflected the popularity of nursing as a career for young, educated women of school-leaving age; despite the low salaries and the limited promotional opportunities, recruitment to nursing remained consistently high and wastage relatively low during the 1970s and 1980s. In their pursuit of improved conditions of employment, nurses in Ireland achieved some success when they procured an improved salary in the late 1970s.

By the 1980s, nurses were becoming more aware of their contribution to the development of the health services and were increasingly conscious of the unique contribution that nurses were making and could potentially make to the care of patients. Informed by international perspectives on the role of the nurse, Irish nurses embraced the ideals of individualised care and the principles and practice of 'new nursing', a perspective that emphasised the importance of nursing assessment and nursing diagnosis in determining the needs of the patient (Fealy, 2002a). The new perspective placed emphasis on the patient's psychosocial needs, and not just the physical needs that arose out of the medical diagnosis; where 'old nursing' was concerned with the completion of tasks related to the medical diagnosis, 'new nursing' took a wholly *nursing* perspective in the organisation and delivery of nursing care (Salvage, 1990; Webb, 1992). The nurse would assess and plan care on the basis of a nursing model of care (as opposed to a medical model), and care would be organised around systems of team nursing and primary nursing (Salvage, 1990). Meeting the needs of the *patient* and not those of the doctor were implicitly at the heart of this new approach.

The nursing curriculum began to reflect this new perspective; subjects like psychology, sociology, communication skills, ward management, and 'conceptual models and the nursing process' received greater attention. In asserting that the nurse had sole responsibility for aspects of patient care, nursing was asserting its disciplinary independence. If 'new nursing' claimed that nursing care should be based on a nursing assessment and a nursing diagnosis, it implicitly claimed that nurses were autonomous and independent practitioners in their own right. By asserting its disciplinary independence, nursing was also implicitly challenging the hegemony of the medical profession, and the idea that nursing was an autonomous profession also implicitly declared that nursing had its own disciplinary knowledge – 'nursing science' – and could therefore legitimately lay claim to a place in the academy (Fealy, 2002a; Hyde and Treacy, 2000).

Into the academy: taking the first steps

In 1975, arising out of concerns that the role of nurses was not clearly defined, that there was a lack of staffing structures, a lack of nursing input into manpower planning, and deficiencies in the training of nurses, the government established a Working Party on General Nursing. Chaired by Brigid Tierney, the Working Party examined the role of nurses in the health service and it considered the education and training requirements for that role. In its Report, published in 1980, the Working Party presented the most comprehensive examination of nursing undertaken in Ireland to that point (Department of Health, 1980). The Report of the Working Party presented a total of 66 recommendations related to the role of the nurse, nurses' grading structures, recruitment and selection, education and training, and the role of the Nursing Board. On the training of nurses, the Working Party pointed to deficiencies in the system of training and, while it considered that student nurses could not be totally relieved of their responsibilities in relation to patient care, it argued that the students' commitment to nursing service should not interfere with their education and training needs. The Working Party recommended that a common basic training for all nurses be introduced; this should consist of a two-year comprehensive, broadly based programme, to be followed by one year of intensive training in the student's chosen branch of nursing. While the changes in the structure of nurse training envisaged by the Working Party were not realised, owing to the financial impact that the changes would have had on the health services, some recommendations in the Report, including recommendations concerning the role of the Nursing Board, minimum entry requirements, and fitness to practise were reflected in the Nurses Act of 1985.

Despite the failure to implement the recommendations of the Working Party in respect of nurse training, the training hospitals were required to introduce major structural changes in the nursing curriculum when the Irish government was required to implement European directives on the training of nurses in 1979 and again in 1991 (Council of the European Communities, 1977, 1989). Each hospital was obliged to provide the student nurse with minimum hours of theoretical and clinical instruction that included instruction in specialist clinical areas like maternity care, paediatric nursing, psychiatric nursing, and care of older persons. The economic impact of the directives was significant in that the training hospitals were obliged to provide a greatly expanded curriculum and they were deprived of the services of their students for up to half of their total training period. Significantly, hospitals could no longer train student nurses on their own terms, but were required to ensure that each student's statutory requirements in respect of training were met. The economic impact of this imperative was so great that the training system, as it was then constituted, had become economically unsustainable (Fealy, 2002a).

Meanwhile, in consultation with the nursing profession in the early 1990s, the Nursing Board had presented proposals for reforming the system of nurse training that were similar to those that the Working Party on General Nursing had earlier proposed (An Bórd Altranais, 1991, 1994). In its Report, *The Future of Nurse Education and Training in Ireland* (1994), the Board recommended the separation of nursing education and nursing service, the introduction of a common core model of training, and the establishment of links with higher education for the purpose of educational validation and accreditation of nursing programmes. The government accepted the broad thrust of the Report; as part of its health strategy in the period, it accepted that it was necessary to 'align the regime for nursing education more closely with the demands of the modern day health service' (Department of Health, 1994a).

The Galway model

Given the government's pronouncement in support of a change in the system of nurse training, the nursing profession in Ireland anticipated change. The anticipated change came in 1994; on the same day that he had formally taken receipt of the Nursing Board's Report on *The Future of Nurse Education and Training in Ireland*, the Minister for Health, Brendan Howlin, announced the introduction of a pilot scheme for a Diploma in Nursing at University College Galway (Simons et al., 1998). Conjointly prepared by University College Galway and the Western Health Board, the scheme provided for the award of a Diploma in Nursing Studies at the point of registration after three years of study, after which time students could opt to enter practice or pursue an additional year of studies leading to the award of a degree in nursing. The scheme conferred full student status on student nurses and, for all but 14 weeks of the three-year training programme, it ended their obligation to work as hospital employees, and it met the training requirements for state registration with the Nursing Board. Running counter to the proposals of both the Working Party and the Nursing Board, the so-called 'Galway Model' did not incorporate a common core element of training for all entrants to nursing, but instead retained the multiple modes of entry to nursing, maintaining the disciplinary distinction between the general, psychiatric and intellectual disabilities branches of nursing.

While it was ostensibly launched as a pilot scheme, the Galway Model was put forward by the Department of Health as the only model for which hospitals and institutions of higher education would receive approval, and this imposition of the Galway Model caused much resentment among training hospitals and their prospective partner institutions in higher education (Fealy, 2002a). Nevertheless, since funding was made available from the Department of Health, and since the Irish Nurses' Organisation would not countenance a two-tier system of training (Madden, 1994), hospitals and third-level institutions took the opportunity that was presented to them and accepted the Galway Model.

The new pilot diploma programme commenced at University College Galway in September 1994. While representing only a partial integration of nursing into higher education, the programme represented the realisation of a long-held goal of nursing to achieve academic recognition for the basic nursing qualification. In the following three years, under the watchful control of the Department of Health, which demanded conformity to a highly prescribed curriculum (Clarke, 1996), the new diploma programme was rolled out at thirteen other universities and institutions of higher education, in partnership with the voluntary hospitals and the health boards. By 1998, recruitment to the traditional hospital apprenticeship-training programme had ceased.

Continuing professional education

The developments taking place in basic nurse training in the 1990s began to be matched by developments in continuing professional education. The area of continuing education had for long been underfunded and there was generally a limited provision to meet the growing needs of qualified nurses who wished to advance their knowledge and skills for new and expanding nursing roles. A survey of nurses in Ireland published in 1999 pointed to the fact that the scope of professional practice had changed enormously, that the role of the Irish nurse was continuously expanding and becoming more specialised, and new roles were emerging for nurses (An Bórd Altranais, 1999). The widening of the scope of professional practice was occurring through changes in the development of the health services and related changes in client needs and through the impetus for professional advancement, which came from within the profession itself. Many nurse specialist roles were linked to medical sub-disciplines such as surgery, endocrinology, oncology and cardiology; some had evolved from medical research assistant roles and there was a lack of clarity between the role boundaries of specialist nurses and medical research assistants (Condell, 1998).

Up to 1995, with the exceptions of a Diploma in Public Health Nursing and a Diploma in Oncology Nursing offered by University College Dublin, post-registration training courses in specialist clinical disciplines were not afforded academic recognition. However, during the early 1990s, there were explicit efforts on the part of employers, the Nursing Board and the higher education sector to bring about increased provision of more coherent, better structured and academically accredited programmes of continuing and post-registration education, and there was also considerable capital investment in infrastructure supportive of the enterprise of continuing professional education. In 1997, the

Nursing Board established an accreditation framework for continuing education and a recording system for post-registration courses (An Bórd Altranais, 1997), while the higher education sector provided flexible modes of study for registered nurses wishing to advance their professional education and training. This included the modularisation of degree, higher diploma and master's programmes, and the establishment of a distance learning degree under the aegis of the National Distance Education Council.

The Commission on Nursing and full integration into the academy

A feature of Irish health care in the last two decades of the twentieth century was the policy of successive governments to rationalise the health services. With the changes that rationalisation brought about, nurses experienced increased workloads and a sense of increasing responsibility, but with no commensurate increase in remuneration or occupational status (Fealy, 2002b). This situation resulted in a period of industrial unrest that culminated in a call for a nationwide nurses' strike in the spring of 1996. The strike was averted at the eleventh hour, with the intervention of the Labour Court, which recommended a salary increase and the establishment of a Commission on Nursing.

The Commission on Nursing was duly constituted in March 1997, and it embarked on a process of consultation and deliberation with and amongst Irish nurses and midwives. Under its terms of reference, the Commission was charged with examining and reporting on such areas as the role of nurses and midwives, promotional opportunities, the requirements placed on nurses in training and in the delivery of service, and the educational requirements of nurses. In making its recommendations, the Commission sought 'to provide a secure basis for the further professional development of nursing in the context of anticipated changes in health services, their organisation and delivery' (Government of Ireland, 1998: 3). The Commission presented Irish nursing with an opportunity to express its views and to suggest policies pertaining to the future of nursing in Ireland (Chavasse, 1998). In its final Report, *A Blueprint for the Future*, the Commission made recommendations pertaining to the regulation of the profession, the educational preparation and professional development of nursing and midwifery in Ireland, and the role of nurses and midwives in the management of services (Government of Ireland, 1998).

On nurses' and midwives' professional development, the Commission recommended the establishment of a clinical career pathway for nursing and midwifery; a clinical career in nursing should advance through the grades of registered nurse, clinical nurse specialist and advanced nurse practitioner, thereby permitting nurses to advance along a professional path that would not remove them from clinical practice. The education and training for the new grades should be pursued through third-level institutions within academic and national accreditation frameworks at the educational level of a master's degree. The Commission also recommended that a National Council for Professional Development of Nurses and Midwives be established; the proposed Council would monitor the development of nursing and midwifery clinical specialities, determine the appropriate level of qualification and experience required for entry into specialist nursing and midwifery practice, and accredit post-registration courses.

Having examined the new diploma programme introduced as the Galway Model in 1994, the Commission adjudged the scheme to have failed to offer the student nurse the full benefits of a third-level education. Citing international trends towards degree-level education for nurses in Australia, New Zealand, Canada and the United States, the Commission called for the full integration of pre-registration (basic) training into the higher education sector, and it recommended that the future framework for pre-registration nurse training be based on a four-year programme leading to a degree in nursing. In its report, the Commission specified the year 2002 as the start-up date for the commencement of the proposed new programme (Government of Ireland, 1998).

Despite the fact that the overall recommendations of the Commission were well received by the profession and were accepted by the government, Irish nurses and midwives became increasingly dissatisfied that long-standing matters related to remuneration for long service and promotional grades and allowances for additional qualifications had remained unresolved. This dissatisfaction led to the first-ever nationwide nurses' strike, with emergency cover, in October 1999. The industrial action lasted for nine days, and its conduct was co-ordinated by a national alliance of nursing trade unions. Support for the strike appeared to be almost total amongst the corps of Irish nurses and midwives, and international support for the action was also forthcoming from nursing representative bodies; the Irish public also appeared to be generally supportive of the nurses.

The industrial action appeared to have achieved its aims; the government expressed a commitment to implement the recommendations of the Commission on Nursing, nurses and midwives received increased remuneration and assurances in relation to long service and promotional grades, and the National Council for Professional Development of Nurses and Midwives was established. While the full story of the strike is outside the scope of the present discussion, the event served to illustrate the fact that nursing in Ireland had gone through much greater change than could be accounted for in educational reform and the expansion of nursing roles alone.

In accepting the recommendations of the Commission on Nursing, the government honoured its commitment to the achievement of the full integration of nurse training into higher education, by providing the necessary funding to permit the establishment of new schools of nursing in the universities and in a number of institutes of technology. This funding included provision for the building of new teaching facilities in the participating institutions of higher education and the transfer of teaching staff from the health services to the higher education sector. In September 2002, the first cohort of undergraduate nursing students entered a new four-year programme and nurse training became fully integrated into higher education. Nursing in Ireland had overtaken many other developed countries, including the United Kingdom, in achieving the status of an all-graduate profession.

Suspicion

While the profession welcomed the move to graduate status, there was evidence that the ending of the traditional system of nurse training was not unconditionally welcomed, either within or outside the profession. When Irish nursing had earlier embraced the ideals of 'new nursing' in the 1980s, at the time, many nurses believed that the only place to study nursing was in the hospital; some were dubious about the clinical capabilities of academically trained nurses or were generally suspicious of the 'intelligent nurse' (McGowan, 1980). When the training of nurses did eventually become located within the academy, hard-pressed clinical nurses and nursing service managers had lost the services of an efficient and compliant worker, the apprentice nurse. Anecdotally, there was evidence of a residue of suspicion among those who still opposed the 'academic' nurse or who were unconvinced of the contribution that a well-educated nurse could make to patient care. However, the profession generally welcomed the development of the new degree programme and it collaborated with the universities and with the institutes of technology in a spirit of partnership to ensure a smooth transition to the new system.

Some in the medical profession in Ireland were less convinced of the need for nurses to be educated to degree level. As early as the 1960s, when there were calls for nurse training to be placed in the academy, some doctors expressed concern that higher education and the higher entry requirements needed would endanger recruitment to nursing, would suppress nurses' 'sense of vocation' and would fail to provide nurses who were clinically competent (Biggart, 1968). Some members of the medical profession were suspicious of the intentions of nursing in seeking degree-level education and viewed the development of graduate-level entry to the profession with some disdain. One doctor criticised the new degree programme, claiming that too much emphasis was laid on academic achievement (Lally, 2002), while another questioned the commitment of the graduate nurse to nursing practice upon graduation, observing: 'Imagine the future frustration of these high-achieving women when reality hits home!' (Tormey, 2003: 47).

The implicit assumptions underpinning these views did not accord with international evidence that pointed to the fact that well-educated nurses remained committed to nursing and to clinical practice (Robinson et al., 2003). These assumptions also appeared to demonstrate a lack of understanding of the nature and/or the function of graduate education for nurses and the benefits that well-educated nurses could bring to the care of patients. Empirical research published in the medical literature demonstrated that hospitals that employed higher proportions of nurses with bachelor or higher degrees in direct patient care had improved patient outcomes (Aiken et al., 2003). The undercurrent of suspicion and resentment at nurses attaining graduate status, which a small number of medical doctors expressed, may have had more to do with an ill-founded sense of threat that the educated nurse posed to medical hegemony, and less to do with any real concern about the quality of nursing care. Commentators like Tormey (2003) also appeared to be visiting many of the ills of the Irish health services on the introduction of the new degree in nursing. Even within the academy, nursing could be understood as a subsidiary activity of medical practice – a 'low rung on the ladder of medicine' – and not understood to be a distinct professional discipline with its own domain of knowledge (Sellers, 2000).

Conclusions

Throughout its first four decades as a modern social practice, nursing's principal project was the procurement of professional regulation. For the four decades following state registration in 1919, a major concern among nurses in Ireland was the improvement in their conditions of employment, including the procurement of pension rights. With the relative economic prosperity that occurred after the 1960s, nurses in Ireland became increasingly focused on their professional education and training and the enhancement of their professional status. After the 1980s, they began to develop nursing scholarship through research and publications in the international academic press. All the while, their conditions of employment were a focus for professional and industrial action, and in common with workers more generally, they began to assert their rights to proper remuneration for their level of skill and responsibility.

A feature of the development of modern nursing in Ireland was its close relationship with the development of scientific medicine and hospital medicine in particular. In the nineteenth century, rapid scientific progress in hospital medicine meant that the doctor needed a skilled nurse to meet the needs of patients receiving prescribed treatments. In consort with hospital medicine, modern nursing developed and matured as a professional discipline, capable of providing skilled care across a range of clinical disciplines and client groups.

Despite its close interdependent relationship with the medical profession, nursing in Ireland began to develop a strong sense of disciplinary identity and a strong desire for disciplinary independence. This desire was articulated in a number of ways, including the efforts to impose perspectives on patient care that were uniquely *nursing*, and in the calls for the reform of nurse training in order to enhance learning and to achieve academic recognition for the basic nursing qualification. The profession eventually achieved the status of a graduate profession at the end of a period of unprecedented economic growth; the financial wherewithal made possible the transition to higher education and, since the 'tiger economy' of the 1990s was coming to an end, the timing was fortuitous.

By situating itself in higher education, nursing had asserted its disciplinary independence and it was redefining its professional relationships with the medical profession (Hyde and Treacy, 1999), with other health care professions, and with other professional groups whose education was located in the academy. As it took its place alongside the other graduate professions in Irish health care, Irish nursing could not expect that stereotypes concerning the educated nurse would dissipate in the single act of entering the academy; public relations alone could not alter attitudes. The benefits that an all-graduate nursing profession could bring would ultimately be demonstrated in the arena of clinical practice. However, through scholarship in the academy, nursing could develop its practice knowledge, express its philosophies and values, and demonstrate its disciplinary independence.

Chapter 7

Learning only to labour

Anne Stakelum

From the 1940s until 1994, an apprenticeship model of training guided student nurse education in Ireland, in which the role of student nurse alternated between that of student and employee. In 1994, following four years of deliberations and consultations between a review body representing nurses, *The Future of Nurse Education and Training in Ireland* report was published (An Bórd Altranais, 1994). The recommendations contained in this report, and later endorsed in the Health Strategy (Department of Health, 1994), advocated changes 'at basic and post basic levels, with the introduction of diplomas and degrees and academic accreditation for all courses' (McCarthy, 1997). This marked the beginning of the end of the apprenticeship model of nurse training in Ireland. By 1998 the apprenticeship model of training was finally laid to rest as all nursing schools had become fully linked to third-level institutions. Radical change has meant supernumerary status for student nurses, where the emphasis now is on education rather than service provision. Students who made up the bulk of the nursing workforce will now be replaced with qualified nurses and other workers. How this newer approach will impact on the profession as a whole and on the student nurses themselves has yet to be determined.

Despite the existence of the apprenticeship model of nurse training in Ireland for over a hundred years, with the exception of Treacy (1987), very little Irish research has been done which explores the process of occupational social-isation from the viewpoint of the student nurses themselves. Their experience of working and learning within the apprenticeship model of training has remained largely untapped in the past, and given the current changes mentioned above, the possibility of revisiting this site for social enquiry in the future is now passé.

The qualitative study described here, using a sample of ten third-year student nurses from two Irish training hospitals carried out in 1994 – prior to the demise of the apprenticeship system – goes some way to redress these gaps in Irish nursing research. Not only this, but it captures the experiences of students socialised within one model of training that can later be used to evaluate newer models of nurse education from the perspective of the student.

Ongoing research into how students view their world of training and work is a necessary tandem to educational and structural changes.

Occupational socialisation

Socialisation has been defined as the process by which individuals learn the culture of their society, both in its more general form and as it applies to particular roles. Student nurses, like other workers at the beginning of their working lives, undergo a process of occupational socialisation where they soon learn the rules and norms of the organisation. According to the functionalist tradition in sociology, these norms define how an individual occupying a particular status is expected to 'act' or behave; roles in a sense provide working lives with order and predictability. Interactionists, on the other hand, argue that roles are often unclear, ambiguous and vague; this lack of clarity gives considerable room for negotiation. Roles, they believe, are not fixed but constructed and negotiated in the process of interaction.

Merton (1957), writing within the functionalist tradition, albeit more flexible than traditional functionalism (Parsons), introduced the concept of 'role set'. This concept is particularly useful as it draws on the notion of 'role conflict' which may occur within the role set and within the multiple roles of a person. Role in this context is a relational term: the nurse plays her role in relation to the counter position of the patient and others in her role set. Merton recognises that the nurse's role enactment (her actual behaviour) may be different from her role demands or prescriptions (her expected behaviour at ward level), and this may not be identical with ideal behaviour (what she should theoretically do). For example, a student nurse is viewed as a learner by her tutor and as a worker by her ward sister, which causes conflict within her role set. This conflict between the educational needs of the student and the service needs of the hospital is further developed by other theorists with varying emphasis.

Professional segmentation theory

Bucher and Strauss (1961) suggest that it is not entirely useful to assume a relative homogeneity within a profession. Rather, they put forward the notion of professions as 'loose amalgamations of segments pursing different objectives in different manners' (1961: 326). Using this definition, then, different segments of a profession may produce different definitions concerning what work should be done and how it should be done (Melia, 1984: 133). In the case of Irish nursing in the past, the apprenticeship model of training was essentially an historical compromise between a services segment and an educational segment in which students were both students and workers. This segmentation meant that the students were under the command of two sets of superiors: the ward sisters representing the services segment, and the tutors representing the educational segment. The professional version of nursing was the one that the nursing school promoted. Its advocates perceived nursing as a 'quasi-scientific' process; in fact it was referred to as the 'nursing process', which took a problem-solving approach to planning and evaluating nursing care (Melia, 1984: 137). On the other hand, those concerned with the provision of the nursing services viewed the 'process' of nursing from a different perspective, more akin to a 'shop-floor' or a 'workload approach'. The emphasis here was less on science and more on getting the work done.

This workload approach, as Melia (1987) suggested, ensured that the work was divided at ward level between various grades of workers: sisters, staff nurses, and students of varying grades. The students were presented to the service as an unqualified workforce and the trained staff found ways of making the system work. Essentially, this meant the 'de-skilling' of nursing work and the subsequent reduction of nursing care into a series of tasks and routines. Students, as Melia suggested, resolve the tensions between both segments by neither learning 'the education segment nor the service version of nursing, but rather they learn to recognise when one version is appropriate and the other is not, and fit in accordingly' (Melia, 1984: 132). This resulted in a compromise between the professional and the service segments of nursing, where students concerned themselves with 'adapting to current situations' rather than preparing in an anticipatory sense to take on the role of trained nurse at a later date.

The study background

Having received permission from the appropriate directors of nursing at two Dublin training hospitals, ten third-year students, five from each hospital, were recruited for this study, which was carried out in July 1994. In the case of hospital A, as the students were dispersed on the wards, working an array of shifts, nominated network sampling was used, the process 'where samples are obtained by eliciting the support and assistance of a single informant already in the study to assist with the selection of another' (Morse, 1991: 130). This proved most appropriate in this instance as it ensured that participating students could not later be identified. This in turn provided for more transparent communication between the student and researcher. In the case of hospital B, as the total population of third-year students was in the classroom at the time of this study, arrangements were made via the principal tutor to speak to the class and explain the purpose of the research. Following this, five students who were willing to participate later contacted the researcher.

Prior to the commencement of the interviews proper, four pilot studies were performed using two neophyte nurses from a hospital not participating in the study, followed by one student from each of the participating hospitals. All interviews were carried out away from the student nurses' working environment, with most of them being done in the students' own homes, or informal settings such as coffee shops.

Generally, what emerged was that while the two nursing schools operated within the same legislative framework, that is they were both subject to the rules and regulations stipulated by An Bórd Altranais (Irish Nursing Board) and within the same structural framework in that all students occupied the dual role of student/employee in the course of their training, differences were found between the ethos and culture of the two environments. These were differences in emphasis, however, rather than fundamental differences. Hospital B differed from hospital A, in that it was more student-friendly and less hierarchical; nonetheless, the same three core themes arose in both hospitals.

Theme one: the student nurse – idealism versus reality

There have been several studies of student nurses and their reasons for seeking nurse training as an occupational choice. These studies, best summarised by Mauksch (1972), suggest that to be needed and to be engaged in personal relationships are the objectives of a majority of nursing students in choosing their career. Furthermore, as Denton (1978) suggests, a person usually chooses an occupation on the basis of images and fragments of information rather than on in-depth experiences within the field. One of the sources of this information is the public image of the field. In nursing this is still predominately the 'surrogate mother image'. For the student nurses in this study the decision to become a nurse was indeed influenced by such an image of nursing. All students chose nursing because they wanted to 'help people', to 'give some of themselves to others'.

This idealised, altruistic version of patient-centred care that the students brought with them to nursing was reinforced in the first introductory 'bloc' [classroom session] the students received. Here their tutors encouraged them to put the patient first. However, in reality when they arrived on the shop floor it was the work that took priority, as this student explained:

> It's a lot different really, I don't think people coming into nursing fully realise what they are coming into . . . it is very different. When you start you think you are going to be there for the patient and you will be able to give him everything, things like that go out the window. Basically with the workload you can't get around to the work you thought you would be doing.

The phase just described is similar in some respects to the first stage of 'initial innocence' as described by Davis (1972) in his description of the six stages of socialisation of student nurses. However, it differs from Davis's account in that the conflict that these students felt arose not because their humanitarian ethic of care and kindness was inconsistent with what their nursing instructors proposed, but rather it was inconsistent with the demands of the training system on the ward which teaches students very early on, that they are first and foremost workers, and 'caring' and affectivity are time-consuming and can be exercised only when the work is done.

Following this initial stage of strain, the conflict the students expressed seemed to heighten to a peak before it reached a plateau. So strong was the conflict between their expectations and their actual experience that some of the students spoke of leaving. Davis has referred to this stage as 'labelled recognition of incongruity'. This was not just confined to the early days on the ward, but recurred at the end of first year and into second year.

While many had felt like leaving, interestingly enough almost all stayed, and out of the total population of all third-year students only one actually left. Student solidarity was the factor they believed had helped them to cope with this period of heightened conflict. This group solidarity, spawned in the early stages of nurse training is a theme that emerges right throughout the students' socialisation period.

Conflict not only revolved around the idealised version of nursing, however, and the reality of nursing work, but it also occurred in the classroom itself where students' perception of themselves as adults and third-year students was at odds with their experience.

Experience in the classroom
As the students' first experience of the nurse training system was in the class-room where they spent approximately 13 weeks, with some supervisory ward sessions towards the end of this period, it was imperative that this area should also be considered. In this instance differences at times quite marked emerged between the two hospitals,

In hospital A, the students felt they were treated as 'children'. While the tutors were often described as 'nice' the lecture format was quite didactic, where students still felt they were being lectured at in a hierarchical setting. This division between teacher and learner was further reinforced by the structural arrangements of the classroom where the furniture was systematically arranged in rows. Time for discussion, whilst it had improved since they were in first year, was far from the ideal of 'self-directive' learning that they had expected.

> I thought it would be different because we were all going to be left school [second level] but it was very much the same, being lectured at and sitting in rows and you

know being given handouts and everything being done for you. Like you don't have to think, you just have to sit there and take notes you don't have to think at all. (Hospital A)

The Nursing Curriculum plays a vital role in maintaining or perpetuating the status quo, or indeed in initiating and facilitating change. While analysis of the actual structure of the curriculum was outside the scope of this study, the accounts of the students suggested a rigid structured series of learning opportunities in which students had to participate in assembly line fashion to be filled with nursing knowledge. It reflects a system that was more like 'an expressway with a one-on, one-off ramp, with little provision for flat tyres, refuelling or sightseeing . . . In an effort to teach the students everything they need to know, the curriculum bulges like an excessively patched inner tube' (Martin, 1990: 566).

In addition, students were quickly socialised into the idea that failure not to grasp what they were taught might some day end up in a disaster with someone dying because of it.

we spent 13 weeks in bloc and basically we were terrified going onto the wards, because we were told if we set a foot wrong we were basically going to end up in court. So we all thought that within six months we were going to be up in court, for something or other. We were there about a week and we were told, that we were the lowest at the moment but don't worry you will have your turn to step up the ladder but it was not put in a nice way. You were made feel so small.

There is no doubt that nursing is a job that involves great responsibility. However, this threat and the atmosphere of fear served to spawn the 'recipient/ object' status on students, who in the hierarchy of things felt powerless. In addition, this approach to the education of students served to promote adaptive rather than change-oriented responses and in doing so served to perpetuate the status quo.

In hospital B the picture was somewhat different. The ethos here was more akin to third-level education, as this student recalls: 'I suppose it is more like college . . . like they give you more or less the skeleton and you go back and it's up to you to look it up for yourself.' Another student commented: 'Basically you are treated like an adult here . . . you are basically in third level now.'

In respect of discussion opportunities, the students in hospital B felt that there was a lot of time for discussion. This depicts a much more student-friendly environment than that described in hospital A and suggests that while both hospitals were governed by the same principles of nurse education, the culture of the hospital itself had a vital role to play in how these were interpreted and experienced by the students. Despite these differences the students' experiences of what they were taught and what they were expected to do at ward level were very similar. All students felt that there was often a lag between theory and practice. These differences had less to do with organisational culture, however, and more to do with the professional segmentation of nurse training. The consequences of this for nurses themselves and nursing as a profession are discussed in the following theme.

Theme two: conflict from occupational segment of training and effects on socialisation

This theme refers to issues that arose for the student nurse as she continually moved between the occupational and the services segment of nursing. In particular it examines the student's experience of the gap between theory and practice: learning only to labour; working in the dark, and peers as educators; flux of responsibility.

Gap between theory and practice
As already mentioned, Bucher and Strauss (1961: 326) suggest that rather than depict professions as a homogeneous grouping it is better to view them as 'loose amalgamations of segments pursuing different objectives in different manners'. According to this concept, different segments of a profession may produce different definitions of what work should be done and how it should be done.

In the case of nurse training, (in the apprenticeship model), two segments could be identified: (a) the educational segment and (b) the service segment. In this study segmentation was recognised quite early on in the student nurse's experience. A 'gap' – to paraphrase their language – existed between the educational and the service sectors of nursing. The school put forward the professional version of nursing, where the status and role of student as learner was reinforced. The ward managers, on the other hand, in the form of staff nurse and sisters, were far more interested in getting the work done. This apparent compartmentalisation, as Melia (1984) also found, created conflict for the student nurse who, by the very organisation of her training, had to cross from one segment into another. These gaps between the educational and services segment of nursing become obvious even in the first eight weeks of training, as this students recalls.

> In PTS [preliminary training school] . . . when we went on to the wards first . . . we'd have an idea of it as they had told us how it was done. But when we went onto the wards the ward staff said: 'well, you are supposed to do it this way. This is how we do it.'

This quotation really captures the dilemma of the student, as she had to cope with the demands of significant others, from either segment – the tutor or the staff nurse. In an effort to cope, students seemed on the whole to sanction the ward way of doing things because it was efficient and it worked, even though it was not entirely correct according to the school of nursing.

This type of 'rule-breaking' is not unique to nursing and has been well documented by Bensman and Gerver (1963), Blau (1963), Ditton (1977) and Melia (1984) who show that 'rule-breaking' is necessary for the smooth running of any work organisation, and if the system is to work new members must be socialised into this legitimated breaking of the rules. Recognising that the hospital is a variegated workshop and not a homogeneous bureaucracy, it was not surprising to find that the degree to which 'rule-breaking' was allowed varied between hospital settings. Busy general wards, where the students were very definitely workers, differed in this respect from specialised wards where the students were often supernumerary. In these specialised units (intensive care, coronary care, theatre), the tensions between the educational and service segment were less acute. Here, students were more learners than workers. This division reduced considerably the 'role conflict' expressed so often by students in other ward settings, a finding which suggests that the current practice of awarding full student status to student nurses has been a move in the right direction.

Learning only to labour

In the course of the interviews students often described a workload that was both physically demanding, but required little real skill. This student in hospital A tells of one of her duties as a third year on her paediatric secondment.

> Some of the wards I was working on the nurse's duty in the afternoon was to start at one end of the ward and work her way through to the other end. There are at least 16 cubicles in the ward and 14 cubicles in the wing, and ... basically you had to empty the bins and the alginate bags [bags for heavily soiled linen] ... I'm not saying that there is anything wrong with it because in the long term maybe it is good training.

Students quickly realised that challenging the status quo at ward level, even if it ran contrary to what they had learned in the classroom, was futile. When asked why she did not challenge issues at ward level that ran contrary to her nurse education, this student put it:

> I think it is because of the fact that you have to get an assessment, the PAF [Proficiency Assessment Form[1]] you know you have to keep your nose clean for these six weeks. You know you have to get a good one.

1   PAF [Proficiency Assessment Form]. This is an assessment of the student's clinical proficiency, given after a student had spent more than six weeks on a ward.

The good nurse was not someone who questioned things but rather one who just did what she was told, as this student recalls: 'The good nurse would be someone who does the work, doesn't ask any questions, doesn't complain or gives out, but just gets on with it.'

How this passivity is institutionalised can be explained when one examines the socialisation of student nurses, from induction forwards. In terms of their hierarchical position, students learned early on that they held a position very low in the hierarchy of things. In the early stages of induction, a sense of powerlessness had already been transferred to the student, one that seemed to grow as she moved through her training. The tasks she was asked to do were often menial and repetitive, but accepted in a fatalistic manner. In addition there was an unwitting acceptance of the experience of relative deprivation as deserved.

On arrival on the wards their sense of powerlessness and inferiority was further reinforced. Students spoke of feeling like 'a plebe' or 'feeling brainless' in this early induction period. They were assigned to a senior student, but all too often, as this student was too busy to show them things, they were left feeling useless. The neophyte nurse soon realised her inexperience was a hindrance to the work ethic on the ward.

> Yes, you were assigned to someone, but then that depended on the ward you were working on. That student could be up and down the corridor and you were standing there and you didn't know what to do. You didn't know the run of the ward. She was so caught up in patient care and she had ten million things to do. They'd say things like 'God I'm really sorry, I know how you feel, I had to go through it. I have to get this, this and this done or the ward sister will shoot me' . . . you sort of stood back then you know because you sort of felt guilty if you were traipsing around after her.

Students learned very early on to 'fit in' with whatever was expedient at the time. They were mainly interested in pleasing those with whom they worked, especially the significant others in their 'role set'. As Melia (1984) found, the students did not see their training from the perspective of either the education or the services segment, rather they saw it as a series of clinical assessments to be got over. The most important thing for them was to get a satisfactory PAF assessment; rocking the boat by over-questioning or being critical of ward ritual served only to prejudice their position. The service sector, therefore, had enormous control over the students' behaviour and they were for the most part preoccupied with learning the ropes on the ward. The balance between the education and service segments was rather one sided, since students eventually realised that they could function on the wards without recourse to nursing pedagogy. Perfecting the ritual and getting to grips with the ward routine was really all that mattered. Professional judgement, therefore, was often displaced with routine and ritual, and skill was attained more by repetitiveness than reason, as this third-year student sums up.

> You could get on without it [bloc/classroom]. I mean the way I look at it, to give a bed bath you don't have to do that by the book. I know like you have to have experience . . . but yet a lot of things you do on the ward a nurse's aid could do as well and she didn't have bloc. She didn't have all these lectures . . . You know she could actually do the same work as you. I mean if she set up a drip four or five times she can do it as well as you can.

In the apprenticeship model of training, in order to facilitate the transition from nursing school to the shop floor, a system of clinical tutors /personal tutors was in operation. The role of these tutors was to provide greater guidance and supervision in the clinical areas. In this study the frequency with which these tutors visited the students varied considerably between hospitals. In hospital A, visits were mainly confined to junior students, while in hospital B all students were visited at regular intervals throughout their training. Despite these differences, tutors were viewed in much the same way by all students: they were a nuisance as they tended to slow down the work.

The question: 'How did you feel when you saw a clinical/personal tutor coming onto the ward?' elicited the following comments.

> Run the other way because she is going to keep you for half and hour and you get no work done. (hospital B)

> I haven't time . . . what does she think I'm doing, does she think I have time to chat you know? (hospital B)

> When I was in first year, I was with a clinical tutor and we took an hour to do a simple dressing. Like I was up to my tonsils in work that morning and I got nothing done. (hospital A)

These comments from the students are reflective of a process of socialisation whereby the work ethic, 'the things', 'the routine', were more important than the reasoning or theory behind clinical practice. So strong was the work ethic, that teaching sessions by the tutor were seen as a waste of time. So if the students saw the clinical tutors as 'a bother' and a hindrance to the work ethic, from whom did they learn? The findings suggest that teaching at ward level was very infrequent, ad hoc and done only when gaps in the service allowed, such as when the ward was quiet or well staffed. Questioning was verbally encouraged but in reality it was tolerated only up to a point. The busier the ward the less time there was for answers. Generally, an ethos of learning was not fostered on the wards; students were essentially seen as 'a pair of hands' to get through the work, as these students explained.

> You'd get fobbed off if it is very busy and you are very enquiring. They'd be going Oh I'll tell you later and casting their eyes up to heaven and that sort of thing.

> I suppose they have too much to do, even if the staff nurses or sisters were more teacher oriented. Like it is a training hospital so you are meant to be learning but a lot of the time you are just a workforce. You are a pair of hands, you learn but it's the exception. It's more hands on that you really learn.

In both hospitals the role-played by the ward sister in this respect was particularly poor. Most of the time she was invisible, or as one student put it: 'You don't actually see sisters, sisters do whatever it is sisters do.' However, there appeared to be some light at the end of the tunnel and it came from the younger, more innovative sisters who in both hospitals had attempted to organise teaching sessions on the ward. Despite these welcome changes, the absence of a systematic link between the service segment and the educational segment of nurse training, and the corresponding poor educational ethos on the shop-floor, meant that students in this study worked mainly in the dark, learning from each other as they went through their training.

Working in the dark: peer learning (1984)
Working in the dark and peer learning emerged as dominant strands running throughout the transcripts. Most of the time the students learned through trial and error, or they learned as they went, getting most information from their peers or newly qualified nurses, who, of all the qualified staff, were the most approachable. These findings cast serious doubts on the nursing education model as it existed prior to the changes introduced after 1994. Not only this but it challenges the very concept of apprenticeship training which is based on the principles of a master/student dyad. Nursing students in this study, unlike medical students described in Becker et al.'s study (1961) who learned from qualified doctors or masters, were not apprenticed to a master as such. This was partly because they were continually on the move between different service segments but more because they found it easier to approach their peers when they needed guidance.

There are serious problems with this scenario, where learners learned from each other, not only for patient care, but also for the development of a student nurse as a skilful, knowledgeable individual, a point highlighted by this student.

> As you go on in your training you do cut corners, sometimes you don't remember how to do it properly which is wrong for a junior student coming on who really is relying on you for guidance.

In addition to learning from each other, students also spent a lot of time working alone and in the dark. The students complained that they were often left short on information about patients' diagnoses. This was partly because the ward report, which all staff members received at the change over of shifts, was short and sometimes inadequate as a working basis. In addition, students were rarely allowed on the doctors' rounds, and as a result not only did they miss out on reasons as to why treatment had been changed but they were often the last to know what changes had been introduced. This non-attendance of students on ward rounds, even as an observer, reinforced the low position of the student in the hierarchy of things; she was a worker whose duty was to carry out routine tasks for which little information was needed as reflected in the following comment

> even the reports vary from ward to ward, in some wards they are very detailed, and they say well he went for this because of this . . . but in many wards you are just told their diagnosis and just told how they were the night before, but you have no indication of what happened in the meantime.

In the late 1980s and 1990s there was an extensive range of articles, particularly in nursing journals, devoted to communication with patients. Nurses were encouraged to talk with patients and adopt a more patient-centred or holistic approach to nursing. However, despite these ideological shifts, the workload approach to nursing in principle still predominated. The ward, at least from the perspective of the student, was seen as the sum needs of 20-plus patients, where caring was seen as a workload to be got through and work was divided on the basis of ability. When asked the question: 'Are you allotted patients, is that the way the system works?', this student responded.

> You'd be given like two wards, like 12 patients and it varies from ward to ward. But you might as well be given obs, temperature, pulse, respirations etc., checking [what] to do, wash them and get them up. You are just doing very basic nursing care.

This task-oriented approach to nurse training not only serves to dehumanise and disempower the students but also to objectify patients who are treated as work objects in the course of the students' routine. The ultimate consequence of this is that patients are precluded from social and psychological care so vital to the recovery process. Furthermore, this approach to nurse training/education harbours serious consequences for nurses themselves, as it denies the development of clinical evaluative powers in the student.

The impact the service segment had on the educational development of the students was further highlighted when one explores how responsibility was transferred to the student as she progressed through her training. For the most part it was not her educational standard but rather the demands of the service that dictated what she was capable of doing. This flux of responsibility was not only frustrating for the students but had implications for the development of their clinical judgement.

Flux of responsibility

Students' accounts in this study suggest that they were exposed to an enormous flux of responsibility in the course of their training. Whilst it varied from ward to ward and day to day, fuelled primarily by varying staffing levels, it was most acute between wards. This was the finding for both hospitals. On some wards the third-year students were treated like junior students, on other wards they were given responsibility over and above what was theoretically expected of them, as this student recalls

> Yes from ward to ward even it's amazing the difference. Like some wards you know you could be left to do the drug rounds, you could be left doing so many things and then in the next ward your responsibility is just squashed again and it is very difficult to cope with.

As upsetting as this continual flux of responsibility was for students, they were powerless to change it. Their acceptance was due not only to the inbred passivity that permeated the whole process of occupational socialisation, but also to the manner in which nurse training was structured. While moving from ward to ward seemed to exacerbate this flux of responsibility, it also served paradoxically to contain it. While one ward might not give them the responsibility they deserved, the next one might; this possibility ensured compliance among students. Related to this flux of responsibility is the notion of transience that permeated the whole process of the apprenticeship model of nurse training. How this impacted on the students themselves is discussed in the following theme.

Theme three: 'always on the move' – the notion of transience

As previously implied, the training programme for students in the apprenticeship model was characterised by students constantly moving from one clinical experience to another, both within and between hospitals and from the college of nursing to the 'shop floor' and back again. During the apprenticeship model of training this transient approach seemed to play a vital role in maintaining the service/education division. In this way the service, it seemed, had an obedient, compliant 'pair of hands' (Melia, 1984: 145). The fact that students were just passing through meant that they would not rock the boat or question a service sector that failed to meet their educational needs. Furthermore, as they were not there long enough to be given any degree of appropriate responsibility, anticipatory socialisation did not occur and thus preparation for the role of staff nurse was impeded.

In this study, most of the students still found moving from ward to ward stressful and upsetting, even though they were now in third year. 'Dreaded' wards were a particular problem. These problems were attenuated somewhat as students learned via informal networks (other students) the do's and don'ts prior to arrival on the wards. While six weeks was the minimum a student had to spend on a ward in order to get a PAF, very often students were moved ad hoc from ward to ward for periods of less than four weeks, which excluded them from any educational feedback. This was particularly noticeable in hospital A, as emerged from these students' accounts

> You are supposed to change wards every six weeks but it was not always possible, with holidays and bloc . . . I mean I was on a psychiatric ward for two weeks before that I was in Temple Street for six weeks, before that I was somewhere else. I'm here for three weeks.

Another student commented: 'Personally I have been changing wards every two to three weeks'. This student believed the reason for such an ad hoc arrangement was: 'I think it is just because of where my name is on the list. My name is on the end of the list . . . so a ward needs somebody. I'm just sent there, a student to make up the numbers.'

Generally, in hospital B, the allocation was six to eight weeks and was more systematically organised. However, most of the students from both hospitals felt that experience on fewer wards and for longer periods (but not too long) would be of more benefit. Most did feel that moving wards was of educational benefit. However, closer analysis of their replies suggests that what students really learned was adaptability, not clinical judgement. Essentially, the opportunity to apply knowledge, identify patterns and recognise the similarities and differences between clinical conditions was limited. This was further highlighted when students were asked if they felt their training had prepared them for the role of staff nurse. With one exception all students felt that they were ill prepared to make the transition from student to qualified nurse; this finding was the same for both hospitals.

> staff nurse is a totally different role in nursing than students. When you qualify you are just thrown in at the deep end and you haven't a clue how to deal with enquiries or deal with relatives. As a student you were always told to call the staff nurse, and then all of a sudden you are a staff nurse and you haven't a clue and nobody's there to show you. (hospital A)

in terms of training, I definitely think students should be trained to be staff nurses and not trained to do students' work. They have to go back and get that into their minds, that they are actually training boys and girls to be nurses. They are not training care workers just to go out and wash people. I know that's part of nursing and part of patient contact . . . but I mean they expect you to do a different job when you are qualified. They expect us to do the paper work, administer drugs . . . the gap is so wide. (hospital B)

In hospital B, on completion of their training, all students were given six months' experience as staff nurses after they had sat their final exams, referred to as 'pre-reging'. In hospital A, very few students are called back for the purpose of gaining experience. While the students in hospital B had a better chance of undergoing some degree of anticipatory socialisation than those in hospital A, it was still unsatisfactory. This arose from the fact that students in their pre-reg period were allocated to the wards not on the basis of their skills or knowledge but rather on the basis of service needs, as this student reveals:

Some days you were counted as a staff nurse. It depends on which member they are short. Other days you are counted as a student nurse.

As the previous accounts suggest, the final transition from student to staff nurse presented a real problem. Until this point, the student's role as worker was mainly concerned with negotiating her way through her placements, adapting as she went. The student had spent three years obediently doing work often of a menial nature in order to obtain the good assessments necessary for her to become a qualified nurse. Through the socialisation process as she moved from ward to ward the emphasis had been on situational learning. When the student was qualified she was no longer straddled between the educational and services sector but firmly rooted in the services sector. In this position she was supervisor of the work, one who allocated the work rather than one who undertook the tasks allotted to her, a completely new experience for which she had minimal or no previous responsibility. One wonders how or when the student was to learn the process of transferring from the routine service version of nursing, to the version of nursing which required astute clinical assessment.

Concern with this transition is reflected in the volume of literature given to the study of changes in values, adaptation and dropout rates in nursing (Hildegarde, 1968; Kramer, 1974; Kramer and Schmalenberg, 1979). Kramer believed that nursing graduates were forced into a situation that they were unprepared for, the process of anticipatory socialisation was not adequately addressed hence the term 'reality shock'. According to Kramer, nurses might respond by dropping out, job-hopping or withdrawing. Given that most of the students in the study did not feel they had been adequately prepared for their role as staff nurses, it is quite possible that they would experience some degree of reality shock in the future. Follow-up studies would be needed, howeverto confirm this. Nonetheless, this piece of research indicated that the students had been socialised into a system where work was divided using bureaucratic principles, where the emphasis was on getting the work done rather than fostering any degree of clinical judgement in the students. Transience, the blueprint of her training, rather than contributing to this process, militated against it. The students were constantly on the move, gaining little of responsibility as the students themselves realised.

> As a student I feel kind of freer, moving around from ward to ward, you know you have no real responsibility in many ways. I feel like . . . moving around, people don't expect you to know the routine straight away, and you are kind of learning again. (hospital B)

In hospital A we get a similar picture. Training was all about passing the buck; in contrast, the world of the staff nurse was about dealing with the buck.

> I mean a lot of nursing is passing the buck. PTS and first years ask the second years, who in turn ask the third years, who pass it on to the staff nurse, and that's where the buck stops.

Summary and conclusions

This study, which looked at the concept of occupational socialisation through the eyes of the student nurse, depicted a process that was permeated with conflict, in particular the conflict the student nurse experienced as she negotiated the educational and the services segment of nurse training. Not only this, but the constant movement of learners, the poor support given to the learner by qualified staff, the pressures of learning and working, and the failure to inculcate critical thinking and confidence in the learners, all point to a system of education that was seriously lacking. Students, while they might learn to perfect routines and rituals, learned little in the way of evidence-based clinical practice. All too often, as Freidson (1970) suggested, deficient behaviour of the professional has tended to be explained as the result of being a deficient kind of person, or at least having being inadequately or improperly 'socialised'. The most commonly suggested remedy in Ireland for such behaviour prior to 1994 was reform of the professional curriculum, rather than reform of the structure in which student nurses were trained.

In more recent times, the professional circumstances of nurse education have changed radically. How these structural changes will impact on the occupational socialisation of student nurses and ultimately on patient care have yet to be determined. One can only hope that it will be inordinately better than the model that preceded it.

Chapter 8

The child health care service: the role of the public health nurse

Margaret O'Keeffe

For the past 150 years, biomedicine has dominated our thinking about health and illness. Biomedicine views the body as a machine, with overriding importance being given to learning about anatomy and physiology and understanding such mechanisms as the heart, arteries, nerves and brain. According to Armstrong (1994: 1), 'it reduces illness to a biological abnormality inside the body'. Consideration of the psychological or social dimensions of illness has little place in such a framework (Weiss and Lonnquist, 1994). The patient was, thus, objectified in physiological realities (Bonda and Bonda, 1986). However, it has now become generally acknowledged that social and cultural factors, not just the physical, influence people's views, reactions and behaviour in regard to health and illness. The emphasis is no longer merely on physical and anatomical changes that occur when one's health alters, but on the whole person, and on his or her social environment. This view has led to the emergence of an alternative paradigm: the social model. The emphasis on a social model is clearly evident in Ireland. An Bórd Altranais (The Nursing Board), in its document *The Future of Nurse Education and Training in Ireland* (1994), states that the delivery of health care encompasses the physical, psychological, spiritual and social aspects of life as they affect health. Kelly (1995: 191) also pointed out that 'public health nursing interfaces with the medical and social models of health'.

The social model, as McCluskey (1997) points out, also recognises the patient as an active participant in the therapeutic process rather than a passive recipient as in the biomedical model. Nettleton (1995: 6) states that those most critical of biomedicine 'have argued that it is essential to recognise that lay people have their own valid interpretations and accounts of their experiences of health and illness. For treatment and care to be effective these must be readily acknowledged.'

It is in this context that social research in nursing proves most useful. One of the central components of current nursing practice is social research. Researchers use a variety of methods in order to gather data, ranging from observation and focus groups to surveys and experiments. Such research yields detailed information about issues of interest to the nursing profession and about the kind of service provided by nurses. The sort of insight provided by research is useful in two ways:

- It provides information on the relation between social factors and patterns of health and illness.
- It contributes to nursing by focusing more on health professionals, helping them to understand how health care can be delivered in a more effective manner (Porter, 1997).

Clamp (1994), described research in nursing as 'providing a link between practice, education and theory, thereby making it essential for all nurses to become knowledgeable consumers [of research]'. Bassett (1992) pointed out that adequate nursing care should, and *must* [my emphasis], be based on a body of knowledge that provides an objective foundation on which nursing actions and behaviours can be justified. Research helps to challenge accepted truths regarding the best methods of health care provision, ultimately providing new ways of approaching health care delivery. Health care professionals must have access to the latest knowledge relevant to their area of expertise, otherwise they cannot hope to enhance the reputation of their profession. Thus, nursing research makes a valuable contribution, providing insights into the perspectives of the patient/client. Bowling (1997: 6) also stresses that 'it is essential to include the perspective of the lay person in health service evaluation and decision-making'. Jones (1994) noted that the idea of the 'the patient's voice' is the product of a particular way of thinking about and viewing the patient, to the extent that the patients are persuaded to 'tell their story'.

In recent years health care professionals on the front line have seen changes in social living which place newer, ever greater, demands on their services. Within the health care professions, a strong emphasis on operating in a 'commercial manner' has arisen, that is, meeting the needs of consumers with due regard to their preferences. As Cowley et al. (1995) point out, the client must remain central at all times. It is in this context that the study discussed here is most useful.

I shall draw on a study conducted in 1995 (McCluskey et al., 1995) at the invitation of the Institute of Community Health Nursing, which sought to investigate consumer perceptions of the child health care services. The study sought to investigate how mothers of infants, up to the age of five, in the Republic of Ireland regarded the services provided to them and in particular how they viewed the role of the public health nurse (PHN). Though the findings were disclosed to members of the Institute of Community Health Nursing, this is the first time that the results have been made available to the general public.

The study involved two stages. Stage one was exploratory, designed to gain initial insights into the child health services provided to children under five years of age, including the services provided to their mothers. The employment of focus groups was the research method considered as appropriate to this part of the study. Focus groups are particularly useful in the exploratory phase of a research project; they are invaluable for obtaining general background information and identifying how respondents conceptualise the areas of interest (Stewart and Shamdasani, 1990). The objective is to encourage involvement and interaction among participants, leading to spontaneous discussion, ultimately resulting in the disclosure of opinions and information (Green and Tull, 1978). In other words, a focus group operates as a sort of 'think tank'. Eight focus groups were conducted in seven of the eight health board regions in the Republic of Ireland.[1]

In the second stage, a survey was carried out in each of the eight health board regions. Mothers were asked in personal interviews to give their opinions on the services available to them and their children. The issues covered in this survey were based on the findings of the focus group reports and on suggestions of public health nurses, representative of all health board regions. A random sample of mothers with children aged one year or over was selected for interview. In all, a total of 387 mothers were interviewed.[2]

Over three quarters of the respondents were in the 25 to 39 year age group, 14 per cent were under 25 and 8 per cent were 40 or over. The median age was 31. Just over one fifth (22 per cent) of the mothers had given birth to only one child at the time of the interviews, one third (33 per cent) had given birth to two children and another one fifth (21 per cent) had given birth to three children. A total of 22 per cent of the mothers had given birth to four or more children. The median number of live births per mother was two. A very small proportion of the mothers (5 per cent) had primary school education only. One third (32 per cent) had a maximum of some post-primary education, another third had completed post-primary level. Over one quarter (27 per cent) had some or had completed third-level education.

In the report which follows it is important to emphasise that the research was carried out in the context of mothers being asked to identify what *improvements* might be made to the child health care services. Most of the mothers' criticisms were aimed at the structure of the services, for example, the

---

1   One health board region was omitted owing to last minute administrative difficulties. Two focus groups were conducted in the Eastern Health Board area, by far the largest in terms of population, of all the health board regions.

2   The focus groups and the survey interviews were conducted by public health nurses, but in all instances the nurses were strangers to the participating mothers.

arrangements for PHN visiting, and the standard or lack of facilities in health centres. Overall, the mothers were high in their praise of the public health nurses and most appreciative of their efforts to provide a high quality service. It is against this background that any criticisms of PHNs must be viewed.

In the analysis which follows the principal findings are discussed under the following headings:

1 views on visiting practices
2 immunisation
3 breast/infant feeding
4 child management
5 mother's health
6 appraisals of health centres

The extracts from the focus groups, quoted below, are representative of comments and views frequently expressed by the participants.

Visiting practices

Generally, mothers in the focus groups were satisfied with the first visit from the PHN, stating that it was very helpful (particularly in relation to a first baby), supportive and useful when a mother might feel isolated or fearful when she came home with her new-born baby. One mother stated: 'Within the first two weeks the PHN visited. Very good and reassuring.' A number of mothers reported that they did not know what to expect, in the sense that they had no knowledge of the actual role of the PHN in relation to a family with a newborn infant. This point is particularly well illustrated by one mother who said that she was 'surprised at visit, did not know the procedures for calling and thought the nurse must be worried, and that is why she is calling a few times'.

Many participants felt also that the PHN's role was one of assessing parents' ability to care for the infant, and that the PHN was investigating for any evidence of abuse. A majority of groups felt that it would be beneficial if the PHN were introduced ante-natally in order to 'get to know the PHN and the services before the birth'. Three suggestions were offered in this regard. First, perhaps the PHN could visit the expectant mother towards the end of her pregnancy. Second, the PHN could work in co-ordination with hospital staff during the ante-natal period. Finally, mothers suggested that a video introducing the PHN in her role would be particularly useful. Such measures, they felt, would prepare and inform them with regard to the duties of, and the services offered by, the PHN.

Mothers felt that it should be normal practice that they were told in hospital that the PHN would be calling, and that the PHN could phone for an appointment beforehand. This would mean that the mother could be prepared. For example, one could make a list of questions, as many respondents ssid that they often forgot to ask certain things during a visit which had occurred to them at other times.

Mothers, then, were clearly in favour of meeting the PHN before the birth of the baby. Such a practice would appear to make considerable sense since it would provide an opportunity for first-time mothers to learn about the work of the PHN, to understand her supportive role and allay fears arising from the mistaken belief that the main concerns of the PHN were assessing a parent's ability to care for her infant and checking for any evidence of abuse. It would also mean that the PHN could visit the mother immediately after her return from hospital rather than having to wait to be notified about the birth of the baby. Significantly, this emphasis on ante-natal introductions complements the strong recommendation of the *Report on Health Care for Mothers and Infants* (Institute of Community Health Nursing, 1983) that public health nurses should be more actively involved in the provision of ante-natal care. It concurs, too, with the proposal of the Institute of Community Health Nursing's *Submission on the Strategy Document: Shaping a Healthier Future* (1994b) that there should be a statutory obligation for public health nurses to visit the post-natal mother within 48 hours of discharge from hospital.

Finally, it was suggested that the first visit should be a 'getting to know you' period, not too much writing to be done or too much information given. There would be more time in subsequent visits for the imparting and assimilation of information: 'The best thing would be for the PHN to call and introduce herself, and then call again when problems have arisen.'

There was considerable agreement that more frequent visits were necessary. Mothers would like the first visit as soon as possible after discharge from hospital, preferably within the first two or three days after discharge and certainly within the first week: 'A visit in the first week is very important, especially with a first baby.' Participants were particularly enamoured of the British system whereby the mother and child are visited every day for the first ten days. Mothers reported that they were frequently too tired to assimilate everything that the nurse was explaining or advising, and consequently they felt that there was a clear justification for more frequent visits, where the mothers had time to talk and feel worthy of the PHN's time.

Mothers clearly valued having a contact number for the PHN as they could phone for assistance when and if a problem arose:

> My nurse did not call as frequently but I knew I could contact her if I had a problem even though she has a big workload. Reassuring to know that I could ring the nurse early and catch her before she went out on calls.

Mothers' views in the survey echoed those of the mothers in the focus groups. Firstly, almost 60 per cent of the 387 mothers interviewed considered it desirable that the mother and the PHN should meet with one another *before* the birth of the baby. It also emerged from the survey that over three quarters of mothers (77 per cent) would prefer that the first meeting take place *at home* rather than at ante-natal classes or in hospital. Secondly, more frequent visiting by the PHN was seen as necessary during the first week of the baby's life; and thirdly, a first baby at all stages of development was regarded as needing more visits than later babies. Most mothers in the survey considered it important that the PHN arrange appointments for her visits – indeed, 27 per cent considered it very important. However, somewhat over one third did not agree.

Immunisation

The Institute of Community Health Nursing (1994a) has expressed its deep commitment to improving the uptake of the immunisation programme and is conscious of the deficiencies in it. This commitment is particularly pertinent in light of the views expressed in the focus groups. The principal outcome on this issue is that the participants expressed a general lack of knowledge as to what the vaccines were for, and which were safe to give to a baby. Such confusion is illustrated by the following comment: 'The doctor asked did I want a three-in-one or a two-in-one – he did not explain the differences.' Mothers were particularly anxious to be informed about immunisation and wished 'to discuss the implications of vaccinations and any side effects'.

A number of groups indicated that they would like to be informed or notified when the child was due for immunisation. In addition, it was felt that parents should be reminded to keep their own record of vaccinations, as they frequently did not realise that they were required to do so. Finally, participants would welcome the opportunity to attend health talks and videos on immunisation at the local health centres.

For mothers in the survey, the best way to learn about immunisation was through direct contact with a health care professional, in most cases with the PHN (54 per cent), but also with the GP (21 per cent). This does not imply that other sources of advice are of little benefit. Information provided by health talks, leaflets, videos and the media, if well presented, can be of considerable value and the issues raised can be further explored in discussions with health care professionals.

Breast/infant feeding

Irish breastfeeding rates remain low compared with the rest of Europe, Canada, America and New Zealand. In the early 1980s the national figure was 33 per cent (McSweeney and Kevany, 1982). Recent figures show that 38 per cent of Irish mothers are breastfeeding when they leave hospital. However, only 26 per cent continue to breastfeed after one month, with 18 per cent exclusively breast-feeding (O'Sullivan, 1999). Respondents expressed wide-ranging views on the issue of breastfeeding. One mother acknowledged at the ante-natal stage that she 'did not know anything about breastfeeding'.

Another mother in the group commented: 'Everyone said it would be great but no one told me about the downside.' Breastfeeding support needs to be more effective before the mother leaves the hospital. Respondents felt that they were not well informed about breastfeeding and the potential difficulties that could arise. Consequently, mothers felt that there was little support available:

> I went to a breastfeeding class in – [one of the principal maternity hospitals in Dublin] before I left the hospital. No one said a problem could arise and to ring such and such a person. I felt there was no one there for me.

Though some mothers felt that the PHN could have been more helpful with regard to breastfeeding, others stated that the PHN was very supportive:

> I was nervous because of first baby, even though I come from a large family who do breastfeed. I found the nurse helpful and it was reassuring to know there was somebody who knew what they were about.

Mothers also expressed annoyance at what they perceived to be too much pressure, particularly in hospitals, to breastfeed. The result of this, according to many mothers, was that those who chose to bottle-feed frequently experienced guilt feelings. The current preference for breastfeeding, as opposed to bottle-feeding, is possibly reinforced by the fact that the World Health Organisation (1989) recommend that all babies be exclusively breast-fed for a minimum of four to six months. In addition, mothers who did breastfeed felt that there was also pressure to breastfeed for a considerable duration. One mother expressed strong feelings on the issue: 'Here in Dublin there is La Lèche [an organisation which helps and supports breastfeeding mothers], but they are over the top about breastfeeding. They feel the child should be breast-fed up to going to school.'

The principal recommendations suggested by the respondents were that special lectures and leaflets on breastfeeding would be useful, and in addition information about breastfeeding groups in their area. A significant number of the focus groups would have liked to see more information and advice on, for example, a mixed diet and spoon-feeding. Mothers expressed a need for more help on feeding from one year onwards and would like the PHN 'to call to the house with leaflets on feeding'. The available literature on this issue sees the provision of advice on nutrition and diet as an important part of the nurse's health promotion role. Nurses are often ideally placed to give advice about dietary changes in relation to health (Mackay, 1995; Wilcock, 1995).

A total of 168 mothers in the survey sample reported that they had breast-fed babies in the past or were breastfeeding at the time of the interviews. It is likely that included here are mothers whose practice of breastfeeding varied from one child to another and mothers who had breast-fed for only a short period. Whether a mother had or was breastfeeding was strongly associated with her educational level – the higher the level of educational attainment the more likely a mother was to have experience of breastfeeding. Mothers with some or complete third-level education were almost four times more likely to have breast-fed than mothers who had, at most, incomplete post-primary education – 78 per cent compared with 20 per cent.

The information from the PHN on breastfeeding and weaning from the breast was considered satisfactory by a majority of the 168 mothers who had breastfeeding experience – just over 70 per cent in both instances. The perception of a minority that 'a lot more' information was required was associated with the mother's educational level: the lower the educational level of a mother the more likely she was to perceive this to be the case.

For mothers in the survey population who wished to breastfeed, easy communication (being available at the end of a phone) and frequent visiting after the baby's birth were the forms of support from the PHN that were most valued. The vast majority of the 387 mothers in the sample appeared happy with the information available to them from the PHN on formulae feeding and on the introduction of solid food; however, one quarter (25 per cent) felt that 'a lot more' information was required on the nutritional value of food. The available literature sees the provision of advice on nutrition and diet as an important part of the nurse's health promotion role. Nurses are often ideally placed to give advice about dietary changes in relation to health (Mackay, 1995; Wilcock, 1995).

Child management

In the focus groups the issue of 'child management' was given considerable attention. Some mothers stated that they did not find books and literature on the subject at all helpful. Others said that they tended to follow them as gospel, which resulted in frustration and annoyance. Consequently, there is, according to mothers who participated in the focus groups, an urgent need for more support in many areas of child management. It was suggested that the PHN could help organise a mother and toddler group in each health centre which would deal with the following areas of concern: teething; discipline; parent-craft for men; hyperactivity; eating problems; behavioural disorders. Two areas, however, appeared to generate most concern. First, mothers felt that sleep problems could be particularly difficult to cope with. One mother told the group that her child had had sleeping problems which she had experienced for a considerable length of time: 'Every night for two years with no support available.' Second, temper tantrums also featured frequently, and created diffi-culties even for experienced mothers: 'On my third child it was very difficult with temper tantrums.'

Again, the survey data were generally consistent with the findings of the focus groups. The aspects of child care in which the advice of the PHN was most valued were sleep patterns, cord care, toilet training and teething. Advice on temper tantrums and on faddy eating – finicky eating or eating without appetite – were also stressed by substantial proportions of the respondents.

Mothers' health

Though generally the work of the PHN was seen in a very favourable light, in one respect some respondents tended to be critical in that they felt that more attention could be given to the mother's health. At the same time a number of groups indicated that they did not expect the PHN to discuss their health as they assumed that she was there just for the baby – the 'baby nurse', as she was referred to. Mothers were also of the opinion that if they had had a pre-vious delivery they received even less attention as it was assumed that they knew everything.

Respondents suggested that more emphasis should be put on the overall psychological health of the mother, as post-natal depression is often exper-ienced. Advice is required regarding support services. This point was supported by the literature available. The 'baby blues' most commonly occurs within the first week after the baby is born, and it is estimated that approximately 80 per cent of all mothers suffer from this in some shape or form which can occa-sionally develop into post-natal depression (Rees, 1995). Foyster (1995) believes that many women will suffer in silence so that the condition can go undetected for long periods of time. In addition, the effects of such depression might have long-term consequences for both mother and child (Murray and Cooper, 1988). Similar feelings were expressed by mothers in the survey population. They placed considerable emphasis on the PHN attending to the health of the mother; this was particularly true in relation to a first birth, but attention to the mother's health was still considered important in relation to later births (table 8.1).

Table 8.1 **Importance of public health nurse attending to mothers' health**

	% Respondents	
	First birth	*Later births*
Very important	81.1	55.0
Important	13.7	25.8
Fairly important	3.1	9.3
Not important	2.1	3.4
Information incomplete	–	6.5
N	**387**	**387**

Source: McCluskey et al. (1995).

The problem of post-natal 'blues' was perceived as a major concern by the vast majority of the survey mothers and they considered it very important that the PHN should discuss this problem with those who had recently given birth. The general emotional state of the mother, incontinence problems and family planning were also considered important topics for discussion. The Institute of Community Health Nursing (1994a) agrees that there is a requirement and a need to identify the health issues of women. This is particularly so, as the PHN is uniquely placed to detect problems such as post-natal depression, or the 'baby blues' in the early stages (Painter, 1995).

Appraisals of health centres

Conditions in some health centres were considered to be very poor. Respondents commented on the fact that buildings were very old fashioned, dirty and unhygienic. These comments are illustrative of respondents' opinions in this regard: 'The state of the toilets is disgusting'; 'Dirty floors for children crawling about and this is a health clinic!' Many respondents also pointed to the lack of facilities in health centres and stated that they were not user-friendly. The main facilities which mothers wanted to see provided were changing rooms, drop-in clinics for advice and, in addition, evening and/or Saturday clinics. To quote one mother: 'There should be evening clinics or clinics on Saturday mornings for working mothers.'

Finally, mothers were in agreement that crèche facilities would be advantageous, as according to one mother: 'It is difficult to visit with small children.' Considerable criticism was also levelled at some health centre doctors. Mothers reported that doctors appeared to be quite rushed and on occasion they were ushered out of the doctor's office while still attempting to dress their baby. To

quote two respondents: 'I feel there is not enough time during visits'; 'I was walking out of the room with the child still undressed.' Another mother complained of the doctor's attitude to her and quoted the doctor as follows: 'The next time you come to the clinic do not bring the toddler along.'

Very high proportions of mothers in the survey population indicated that their health centres were unsatisfactory in respect of crèche facilities (92 per cent) and baby changing rooms (78 per cent), probably because in most cases such facilities were not available. Sizeable minorities were critical of toilet facilities (28 per cent), general maintenance (28 per cent), ventilation (28 per cent) and easy access to the building (25 per cent). But the overwhelming majority reported staff courtesy as being very satisfactory or satisfactory (89 per cent). When the mothers' overall rating of their health centres were analysed it emerged that most were reasonably satisfied – indeed, a substantial proportion (40 per cent) gave their centre a high rating. However, a strong association was found between the mothers' level of educational attainment and the overall rating of their centre – those with higher educational levels were more critical. Over one third (35 per cent) of those with some or complete third-level education gave their health centre a score of four or less out of 10 (table 8.2).

Table 8.2 **Overall rating of health centre by level of mothers' educational attainment**

	Ratings 0–4	*5–7*	*8–10*	*N*
	%	%	%	
Primary education only/				
some post-primary education	16.2	33.8	50.0	142
Complete post-primary education	21.9	36.7	41.4	128
Some or complete third level	34.7	37.8	27.6	98
N				**368**

Source: McCluskey et al. (1995).

Discussion

The main question addressed in the analysis which follows is whether the operation of the present-day child health care services represents a major shift from a biomedical to a social model of health and illness where mothers are encouraged to be active participants in decisions relating to themselves and their children or whether, on the other hand, a predominantly asymmetric relationship still persists between the service providers and their clients.

The biomedical model posits the idea that all disease can be understood in biological terms, stressing the importance of scientific knowledge and technical expertise. Until recently, nursing manuals emphasised the need for detachment and objectivity, focusing on the patient's physical needs (Jones, 1994). Today, the role of the nurse is by no means a single, well-defined set of rights and obligations. The focus has altered to the degree that care-giving is now more holistic, with an emphasis on client-centred practice.

The mothers' expectations of the PHN's role are clearly situated within the social model of health in which the emphasis is on patients as 'bio-psycho-social wholes'. This is manifested in the mothers' views that the PHN should attend to the physical, social and psychological health of mother and child. They do not see the role as confined to purely medical issues. Mothers in the study expected PHNs to take account of the social conditions and lifestyles of their patients, their psychological well-being and not just their physical health. According to Robinson (1978), this shift to a more expansive role may be partly explained by the fact that with opportunities for close personal contact lessening and populations becoming more geographically mobile, problems which were hitherto handled by family and community are increasingly being transferred to the formal health services. Brearley et al. (1978) make a similar observation. They note that in the earlier part of this century, there was a surplus of single women who cared for children, the elderly and the infirm. This, they argue, is no longer the case. Today, changes in family structure coupled with increasing numbers of women in the labour force have resulted in a reduction in the supportive network provided by the extended family.

During the 1960s, the concept of the individual as 'consumer' was established (Reeder, 1972). In the age of consumerism, the social role of the health professional could not escape modification (Cockerham, 1995). As we have already seen, role expectations have changed from those envisaged by the biomedical model. Additionally, the belief among lay persons that the 'doctor knows best' is no longer accepted (Cassell, 1986). The notion of the individual as consumer creates a more equal basis of interaction. In particular, individuals are seen as having an input in their own treatment (Strong, 1977) and are encouraged to voice their views on the quality of service. As Nettleton (1995) notes, those who use health care services are being encouraged to exercise their choice and act as discriminating consumers. Oakley (1993: 55) points out that 'people who "buy" products and services . . . must be respected by those who sell such things'.

There is clearly a move towards a consumerist attitude among mothers in the study. They were critical about a number of dimensions of the child health services provided. More frequent visiting, improved standards of care, the availability of additional facilities in health centres, and more attention to the mother's health were identified as requiring urgent attention. The level of criticism directed at health centres is particularly pertinent given that the health centre, according to Woods (1978), has been considered an essential element of good primary care for a considerable time. The inadequacy of health centres has been highlighted elsewhere. The Institute of Community Health Nursing (1994a) noted that various organisations have repeatedly highlighted the poor conditions of health centres. The primary objective in improving such centres should be to ensure that they are 'user-friendly', with an emphasis on meeting consumer needs in an effective manner. Nettleton (1995) argues that women are likely to hold strong views about the health practitioners with whom they come into contact, given that they frequently act as providers and negotiators of health services for others. Strong (1977: 39) noted that there is a 'discrepancy between the desires of patients and their ability to control medical encounters'. This generates feelings of helplessness and frustration resulting in complaints about lack of control which are frequently voiced in consumer satisfaction studies. The patient's time with the doctor is not theirs at all. It is at the doctor's discretion. Doctors, however, often identify a shortage of time as the main constraint on embracing patient-centred approaches (Scambler, 1997b). For them, each case is part of a day's work and schedules are easily disrupted by other contingencies (Strong, 1977).

Zola (1978: 254) has argued that medicine is a major institution of social control: 'It is . . . the new repository of truth, the place where absolute and often final judgements are made . . . in the name of health.' Nettleton (1995) agrees, suggesting that the control of physical bodies by the medical profession is in the ascendant. A central concept which runs through the work of Foucault is that of *disciplinary power*. This concept refers to the way in which human bodies are observed, controlled, regulated and understood. One of the sources of disciplinary power is the medical profession. Foucault (1979) discusses three main aspects of disciplinary power. The first is *hierarchical observation*. This refers to locations where individuals can be observed. Information is collected and collated. This requires what Foucault (1980) calls an 'inspecting gaze' which causes those under its weight to exercise control and surveillance over themselves. The second aspect of disciplinary power is *normalising judgement* which refers to the notion that individuals are compared, resulting in the establishment of norms or accepted standards of behaviour. Health care professionals are but one group capable of exercising judgement. The final aspect discussed is the *examination*. This permits inspection and treatment in an effort to correct abnormalities. Again, the examination is carried out by health care professionals, among others. Medicine's control extends to healthy people in the form of preventive care and adopts a normative posture distinguishing between the healthy and the unhealthy (Ritzer, 1996). Through observation, judgement and examination, health professionals amass knowledge which generates a basis of power. As Ritzer (1996: 599) notes, Foucault 'sees knowledge generating power by constituting people as subjects and then governing the subjects with the knowledge'. In essence, he sees the medical professions as exerting power through knowledge. They have access to a wide range of information which is not usually at the disposal of their patients/clients. In this way, they have the ability to exert influence and ultimately power over those who require and seek their services.

Do the services provided to mothers and their babies constitute a form of social control and, if so, do mothers accept it or not? There is evidence in the study to suggest that child health services exert or attempt to exert considerable control and influence over mothers and their approaches to motherhood, particularly in relation to breastfeeding and hospital immunisation. Mothers expressed annoyance at the pressure to breastfeed, particularly in hospitals, and felt that there was a lack of information on the subject. They implied that potential problems were kept from them and those who did not breastfeed, or who had difficulties, were made to feel that they were not fulfilling their maternal role adequately. It has been argued elsewhere that the institution of medicine dictates what it considers to be appropriate social roles for women and thus, notions of 'womanhood' (Elston and Doyal, 1983). This argument is relevant when looking at breastfeeding. It clearly relates to Foucault's notion of normalising judgement. Health care professionals and organisations establish normative standards against which we are compared. In this case, breastfeeding is considered the norm for new mothers. Mothers felt that they were being judged if they did not or could not breastfeed. They were not conforming to accepted notions of motherhood. In other studies (Kirkham, 1983; Hart, 1985), patients also expressed dissatisfaction at not being kept informed about health-related issues. This point has been made by Byrne and Long (1976), who suggested that doctors deliberately kept patients in a state of ignorance by employing a strategy of information control. This is an argument made also by Foucault. However, while the withholding of information can be a method of exerting control, it is also likely that information and support may serve to determine whether mothers continued to breastfeed. Rajan (1993) found that information and support from health professionals were positively related to the decision to breastfeed. In an Irish study, Wiley and Merriman (1996) asked mothers what would have helped them to continue breastfeeding. Over ten per cent of mothers said that more encouragement from the nurse or health visitor would have been crucial in their decision to continue breastfeeding.

In health prevention, the 'extension into life' becomes even deeper, since the very idea of primary prevention means getting there *before* the disease starts (Zola, 1975: 176). In this way, medicine functions as an institution of social control. Immunisation is one of the principal methods of primary prevention and could therefore be considered a form of social control. All mothers are encouraged to have their children immunised, and the mothers in this study were no different in that regard. The benefits of immunisation are constantly expounded by health care professionals. Gustavsson and Segal (1994) argue that immunisation is vitally important for young children as it is one of the best ways to safeguard them from preventable disease. The Institute of Community Health Nursing (1994a) has also expressed its commitment to improving the uptake of the immunisation programme. However, many mothers in the study felt that they were not sufficiently informed about the vaccination services including whether or not there were likely to be any side effects for the child. This lack of knowledge left mothers often confused and from the discussions in the focus groups it appeared quite clear that many did not experience any sense of personal control when participating in the immunisation programme.

Finally, quite a few participants were under the impression that the PHN's role was primarily one of assessing parents' ability to care for the infant, and that the PHN was therefore checking for evidence of abuse. Again, Foucault's concept of hierarchical observation is evident here. Many mothers felt that they were being monitored and observed and that they came under an 'inspecting gaze' which emanated from the PHN. This made them feel as though their parenting skills were being judged and assessed.

The important implication from the findings is that mothers were not prepared to accept the services in an unquestioning manner but were anxious to be well informed about them. It is also important to note that our knowledge about health and illness is obtained from medicine owing to the fact that it has secured a position of influence, ensuring that its version of what is good for our health becomes *the* orthodox version (Hart, 1985). It is also noteworthy that as patients/clients move towards a more social and holistic health model, and as health care professionals delve into the social and psychological aspects of health, the effect will be to widen the surveillance and power of the profession. The implication is that all areas of the patient's existence will be open and subject to surveillance, observation, judgement and examination, not just the physical (Porter, 1997). Whilst one may conclude from this that the medical profession establishment will retain, and build upon, its current power base, the rise in a consumerist orientation amongst its clients may increasingly act as a counterbalance to this, thus altering the power relations between both parties.

Part 3

The doctor–patient relationship

Chapter 9

The changing face of general practice: the role of the family doctor

William Shannon

From the early days of its foundation in 1952, the Royal College of General Practitioners (RCGP) (UK) attracted to its membership many Irish family doctors who espoused its aims 'to foster and encourage the highest standards in general practice'. Throughout the 1960s, 1970s and 1980s, several hundred Irish general practitioners (GPs) became members of the Royal College until the establishment of the Irish College of General Practitioners (ICGP) in 1984. Even then, and up to the present day, some Irish general practitioners still take the membership examination of the RCGP (MRCGP) even though they also may sit and pass the equivalent examination of the Irish College (MICGP). Although the two examinations differ in detail the standards are regarded as equivalent. Nevertheless, reciprocal membership is not allowed; it is necessary to pass each examination independently before being eligible to become a member of the respective college.

The year 1984 was a milestone for Irish general practice, and with the vision and single-minded energy of its first chairman of Council, Dr Michael Boland, the College has gone from strength to strength in less than 20 years. It has over 90 per cent membership of all Irish general practitioners and an impressive output of publications covering several aspects of general practice development, including vocational training, continuing medical education, practice management and research. In addition, the ICGP has played an active role in helping to establish a department of general practice in each of the five Irish medical schools in the Republic of Ireland, and is committed to supporting them through its members.

The Royal College of Surgeons in Ireland was the first of the Irish medical schools to establish an independent chair and department in 1987. This was indeed another milestone for Irish general practice and made a statement to the medical profession, the Medical Council of Ireland and the other four medical schools that general practice was a discipline in its own right and deserved to be involved in undergraduate medical education and research, as well as in its more established role of vocational training and continuing medical education. Soon after, the other medical schools responded, first with University College Dublin creating a chair of general practice in 1991, then Trinity College, Dublin in 1993, University College Galway in 1996 and finally University College Cork in 1997.

European definition of the general practitioner

In 1974 a group of enthusiastic and academically minded general practitioners met at Leeuwenhorst in the Netherlands and agreed the following definition as being applicable to what a general practitioner's role would be in Western Europe. This definition has achieved wide acceptance and is introduced here as a starting point to help readers recognise the general practitioner as being the most widely available primary health care doctor in the community. The masculine gender was used throughout this quotation in a document written many years ago:

> The general practitioner is a medical graduate with specific training to give personal, primary and continuing care to individuals, families and a practice population, irrespective of age, sex and illness; it is the synthesis of these functions which is unique. He will attend his patients in his consulting room and in their homes and sometimes in a clinic or hospital. His aim is to make early diagnoses. He will include and integrate physical, psychological and social factors in his considerations about health and illness. This will be expressed in the care of his patients. He will make an initial decision about every problem which is presented to him as a doctor. He will undertake the continuing management of his patients with chronic, recurrent or terminal illnesses. Prolonged contact means that he can use repeated opportunities to gather information at a pace appropriate to each patient, and build up a relationship of trust which he can use professionally. He will practice in co-operation with other colleagues, medical and non-medical. He will know how and when to intervene through treatment, prevention and education, to promote the health of his patients and their families. He will recognise that he also has a professional responsibility to the community. (Leeuwenhorst Working Party, 1974: 117)

In the discussion which follows the terms 'general practitioner' and 'family doctor' will be used interchangeably.

Principles guiding the family doctor
McWhinney (1981) has given nine guiding principles of family medicine to which I have added a tenth, covering the important role of the family doctor as advocate for his patients. Whilst these are not unique to family medicine they

are recognised as core values exemplified by a majority of family doctors working in Ireland and Britain.

1 *The person will take precedence over the disease.* This principle puts the person at centre stage and acknowledges that it is legitimate for people to present to their family doctor with any problem and not just a medical one. In other words, the person coming to consult the doctor defines the problem, without necessarily medicalising it. Allied to this is the fact that the family doctor undertakes to give ongoing commitment, and will not be limited by one episode of illness.

2 *The doctor will focus on understanding the context of illness,* which in turn should lead to a fuller understanding of the person as well as the possible disease process, and the steps needed for resolution of the illness.

3 *The doctor will focus on more than the presenting problem* and thereby use opportunities for patient education and prevention.

4 *The doctor will view the individual and the practice as a whole at one and the same time,* for example, a child coming for an acute medical problem will have his/her file checked to ensure the immunisation schedule is up-to-date. I call this practice 'adjusting the lens' so as to focus on both the individual and the practice population during the same consultation opportunity. Others have described this as 'opportunistic care'.

5 *General practice will be seen as part of a community-based network of caring facilities or agencies.* Ideally, all such services would be closely co-ordinated under one roof, but in Ireland a number of factors combine to frustrate this. One major factor must be the two-tier system of general practice whereby two thirds of the patients must pay their family doctor for all consultations, whilst one third are covered by the state-sponsored General Medical Service scheme (GMS). One important consequence for the private, fee-paying sector is that the family doctor feels constrained in offering preventative medicine consultations which will incur a fee each time. This does not happen in the case of the GMS sector, where the patients have free access to the family doctor and to related services, such as those of the practice nurse and public health nurse.

6 *The family doctor will be recognised as a member of the local community.* This is the situation throughout the length and breadth of rural Ireland, where 52 per cent of general practitioners work single-handed and live in or near their practice population. It is less true of city-based general practitioners who often live several miles from their place of work and who therefore miss out on gaining a full understanding of the problems arising in a local community, of which they are not a part.

7 *The general practitioner may see patients in any one of three settings depending on circumstances.* Most consultations will take place in the general

practitioners' consulting rooms or surgery premises; less often, patients will be seen in their own homes and on a few occasions may receive attention in a local or district hospital, if their family doctor has visiting rights there.

8 *The general practitioner will pay due attention to patients' feelings*, especially their fears and anxieties, which may have either caused or precipitated any one of a variety of illnesses.

9 *The general practitioner will act as an advocate for his or her patients.* In a time of increasing complexity of medicine and especially technology the central role of the family doctor as *patient advocate* has become even more important today. Lay people are being bombarded with new information in the media, especially on TV and the Internet, and will commonly consult their trusted family doctor for guidance in sifting through the maze while trying to find an appropriate solution for their health care problem. This role has major implications in relation to the need for the family doctor to keep up to date.

10 *The general practitioner will act as a resource manager.* This final role of the family doctor has become increasingly important in recent years with the enormous rise in health care costs and the need for governments and funding agencies to control them. As the principal first-contact physician, the general practitioner can incur add-on costs in three main areas, namely prescribing, investigations and referral to secondary care specialists. By far the most expensive of these activities is referral, although most of the studies to date have centred upon the more measurable area of prescribing, where there is already evidence of cost-savings without any apparent loss in either doctor autonomy or quality of care for patients.

In the case of prevention, there is abundant evidence that the *practice nurse* (see below) has a key educational and preventative role which Irish general practitioners are rapidly recognising as being a core part of good general practice, and not just ancillary to it. Twenty years ago there were no more than a dozen or so nurses working in Irish general practice; in 1998 that figure had exceeded 400 and is rising, as the value of having a nursing colleague working in general practice is fully realised by health boards and family doctors alike. The General Medical Service contract of 1990 gave a significant fillip to the employment of practice nurses by offering general practitioners the incentive of partial reimbursement of their salaries proportional to the size of their GMS lists.

The discipline of practice management is only starting to be appreciated in Irish general practice. With the continued emphasis on achieving value for money and accountability it is clear that all general practitioners will need basic practice management skills to survive financially. Those working in group practices will likely turn to professional managers for their expertise and skills in terms of day-to-day practice management and the further development of the general practice as a whole. Practice managers have represented a key part of British general practice for many years. There, the general practitioner is very much part of a multi-disciplinary team, with a suitably trained practice manager who works in close association with the partners. This arrangement enables the doctors to conserve their time and energies for their clinical work, while the practice manager gets on with the business of running the practice. Even if we in Ireland continue to have roughly one-third GMS and two-thirds private practice, it will become increasingly obvious that good standards of clinical practice depend on good time and practice management, so that all personnel can achieve their maximum potential as a team, rather than as a collection of individuals.

Development of the patient-centred interview

The French appear to have been first to write about the doctor/patient interaction and to present to the world a very doctor-centred model of the consultation. The American sociologist, Talcott Parsons (1951), devised a very elegant model of the doctor–patient relationship which proposed that the roles of doctor and patient, like other social roles, consist of both rights and obligations. He argued that the relationship entails a basic mutuality, each party – the doctor and the patient – was expected to be familiar with his or her own and the other's expectations of behaviour. However, Parsons conceived of the relationship as being very much an asymmetric one. He saw professional dominance as inherent in the doctor's role. The patient was assumed to take a dependent and subordinate posture in many, if not most, of the interactions between the two parties.

In more recent times there has been a palpable shift to a more patient-centred approach which is inclusive of the patient's as well as the doctor's agenda. One might add that the doctor-centred approach has also been a very biological one with its focus on the search for organic disease, while the more inclusive patient-centred approach is often described as being *biopsychosocial* (Engel, 1977). This means that the doctor will give due attention to the psychological and social factors in a patient's presentation of illness and not merely be confined to looking for organic disease.

Pendleton and his colleagues (1984) have arguably made the single greatest contribution to our clear understanding of the tasks and processes involved in doctor/patient interactions. They have summarised the seven tasks of the consultation or patient-centred interview as follows:

1   To define the reasons for the patient's attendance in physical, psychological and social terms: nature and history of problems; aetiology; patient's ideas, concerns and expectations; effects of problems on the patient and/or family.

2 To consider other problems: continuing problems; at risk factors.
3 With the patient to choose an appropriate action for each problem.
4 To share the doctor's understanding of the problem with the patient.
5 To involve the patient in the management and encourage him/her to accept appropriate responsibility.
6 To use time and resources appropriately: in the consultation; long term.
7 To establish or maintain a relationship with the patient which facilitates the achievement of the above tasks.

I like to emphasise to students of family medicine that there are three distinct phases to the consultation. The most evident is the interview itself but the other two are equally, if not more, important in determining outcome. These latter are what are known as *the pre-consultation phase* and *the post-consultation phase*. The pre-consultation phase acknowledges the fact that patients and their doctors, especially family doctors, have a certain amount of foreknowledge of each other before the actual interview or consultation takes place. The doctor may know the patient for many years, and may have treated him/her in the past, and therefore be in possession of a lot of information prior to the consultation. This background information will normally speed up the process of consultation since the experienced doctor has learned how to focus on the patient's principal problem before agreeing the most effective line of further investigation or treatment. At the same time, the patient will also have foreknowledge of the doctor, whom he or she may know for many years. Regardless of the circumstances or background knowledge, the patient will usually have certain fears or anxieties before consulting and will also have expectations about what might happen during the consultation. These expectations and fears may have been coloured by the patient's discussion of his or her problems with family or friends, since very few people consult the doctor without being influenced by either past experience, personal fears and/or advice from a friend or family member. If the pre-consultation phase is an important component leading up to a consultation then the post-consultation phase is equally important since it represents the outcome of the patient/doctor inter-action. An effective consultation will largely determine the level of compliance of the patient. It is the doctor's obligation to ensure that the patient has been fully involved in the consultation process and has clearly understood what his problem is and what needs to be done to resolve it.

Levenstein et al. (1989) have given a clear model for effective patient-centred interviewing. They point out that while medical people have a well-defined traditional clinical method for interviewing, aimed at diagnosing and under-standing diseases, we have no equivalent method for understanding patients as people. It is my firm belief that it is often more important to understand the person who has the disease, than the disease the person has.

Figure 9.1 **The patient-centred clinical interview**

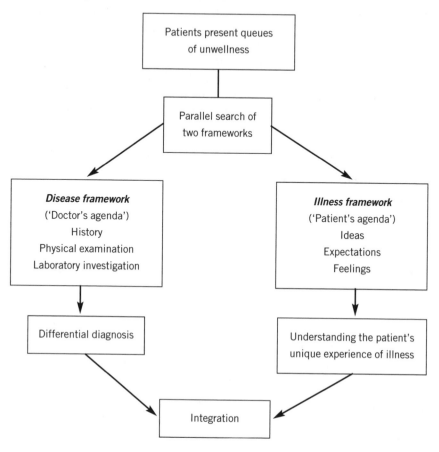

Source: Adapted from Levenstein et al. (1989)

In the relatively new, patient-centred approach, the physician's aim is twofold. First, the doctor must attend to the patient's agenda. This involves trying to understand the patient's expectations from the visit or interview and in particular to ascertain the role of feelings, and especially fears, in causing him or her to consult in the first place. Next, the doctor needs to ascertain their expectations from the visit or interview and then to focus on the specifics to confirm or exclude a disease process, by reference to what is termed the doctor's agenda. Following this agenda means the doctor traces the development of any symptoms and physical signs, in order to clarify whether they represent a pattern that is recognisable or warrants further investigation or, as in many cases, is not indicative of serious disease. Even in the absence of any serious disease, there is still a requirement on the doctor to come to an understanding of the level of dysfunction which might require modification of a patient's life-style, or some other action on the patient's part, rather than medical or surgical action on the doctor's part.

Many years ago, Szasz and Hollender (1956) gave a model of the doctor/patient interview which regrettably did not then lead to the changes from traditional medical paternalism that they had probably hoped for. Their model was intended to make explicit the evolution from patient/doctor dependency to mutual or adult/adult participation. Their three-part model, which moves from activity–passivity, through guidance–co-operation to eventual mutual participation is summarised in table 9.1.

Table 9.1 **Szasz-Hollender models of the doctor–patient relationship**

Model	Physician's role	Patient's role	Clinical application of model	Prototype of model
Activity–passivity	Does something to patient	Recipient (unable to respond or inert)	Anaesthesia, acute trauma, coma, delirium.	Parent–infant
Guidance–co-operation	Tells patient what to do	Co-operator (obeys)	Acute infectious processes.	Parent–child (adolescent)
Mutual participation	Helps patient to help himself	Participant in 'partnership' (uses expert help)	Most chronic illnesses, psychoanalysis.	Adult–adult

Source: Szasz and Hollender (1956: 586).

In Irish medical schools today, teaching communication skills leading to an understanding of what takes place in the consultation is included in all curricula, though it is still largely the remit of the departments of general practice, rather than being fully embraced by the medical school faculty as a whole. Academic general practitioners and psychologists are working to bring about a greater degree of self-awareness in medical students and family doctors in training, as a prelude to enhancing their effectiveness in coping with patients and families, whose problems are often as much psycho-social as strictly medical.

The contribution of general practice to a medical school and medical education

Studies both in Ireland and in the UK have confirmed that 90 per cent or more of all illnesses and problems presented to the family doctor are managed by him or her, without referral to secondary care or the hospital system. In an audit of my own practice published in 1983, my referral rate to secondary care was nine per cent per annum (Shannon, 1983). The Irish College of General Practitioners has found that the referral rate can be even less, of the order of four or five per cent. What this means is that many of the problems and illnesses, including important common conditions such as anxiety and depression, rarely get to hospital, except in their more severe forms. The fact that such a huge percentage of morbidity is dealt with solely in the general practice setting means that medical students miss out on the bigger picture when most of their clinical training is at the highly concentrated hospital end of the spectrum, as distinct from in the community.

In 1988, at an international conference on medical education hosted in Edinburgh by the World Federation for Medical Education, one of the main concerns was the need for more community-based teaching. The departments of general practice in the Irish medical schools are now responding, in so far as curricular time and teaching resources allow, but there is still much to be done towards closer collaboration with other disciplines, to achieve an integrated curriculum, rather than being either subject or department based. Placing students in the community or general setting provides them with first-hand experience to enable them to make an informed career choice. This is especially relevant when we know that in Ireland over 50 per cent of any final year medical class will opt to be trained as family doctors. The overall aim of a general practice student attachment in Ireland is to introduce the student to the principles and practice of clinical medicine in the setting of the community via the general practitioner or family doctor. It is not the intention in any way to train the student for general practice, which is a postgraduate discipline requiring three or four years' special training after registration as a doctor. Indeed, the belief is that, just like many of the departments of general practice in the UK medical schools, experience in general practice and the community is even more important for those students who will specialise in hospital medicine, so that they can fully understand the context from which their patients come, and to which they will return.

Another significant message from the international conference in Edinburgh was that medical education itself should become less dependent on the traditional lecture, which fosters passivity, and become more student-centred and active, thereby fostering the concept and practice of lifelong learning. The parallel to this in general practice is the patient-centred approach which, as described earlier, forms the keystone of much of our teaching in the general practice setting. This is done through a combination of one-to-one teaching in the practice and also in the small group format, with a tutor/facilitator leading a small group for communication skills and consultation analysis work. Another important lesson from the Edinburgh conference, which is of central importance to all medical schools, was the need to make learning more problem-based rather than just learning by rote or about science in the abstract. An important part of our family medicine teaching uses modified essay questions, which are essentially unfolding, problem-solving exercises with an emphasis on the students working in small groups to tease out the options for resolving common clinical problems. Computer-assisted learning is also being developed, with the aim of fostering interactive small group learning, which the students greatly enjoy. The discipline of general practice has also made a special study of medical education, particularly in the area of the training of examiners. Much pioneering work in this area was developed by the Royal College of General Practitioners in the UK, and more recently by the Irish College of General Practitioners. Both of these institutions have learned much from the disciplines of education and psychology in order to inform their members about the impor-tance of specific training for examiners in the vital work of both formative and end-point assessment. The Royal College of General Practitioners in the UK was the first such institution not only to provide formal training for its exam-iners, but also to monitor their performance at intervals to ensure consistency and reliability over time.

Lifelong learning: continuing medical education or continuous professional development?

For many years, hospital specialists have seen it as part of their duty or obligation to update general practitioners on new developments of relevance to them. It was assumed that if there were developments, particularly of a tech-nological nature such as new techniques in surgery, then general practitioners ought to know about them. It was also assumed by the general practitioner that the best, if not the only, people to teach them were the hospital specialists/consultants. *Teach* was the operative word since it was also assumed by both parties that the best way to get a message across was to tell somebody, even if it was not a priority need for the busy general practitioner. The sponsors of such educational meetings, principally the pharmaceutical industry, were also included in this exercise, under the banner of continuing medical education (CME), in the hope that GPs would turn up in sufficient numbers to justify their investment. All that has changed for the better in recent years due to the combined efforts of both the Royal College of General Practitioners and the

Irish College of General Practitioners. Initially it was shown how general practitioners could learn a lot from each other, once they had been given some ideas on how to capitalise on the wealth of clinical material arriving on their surgery doorsteps each day. They could do this in an orderly way once they also learnt some key educational principles and techniques borrowed from other disciplines, especially educational psychology. Later, following the establishment of the Irish College of General Practitioners, Michael Boland showed Irish general practitioners how to utilise their own resources with the establishment of a nationwide network of continuing medical education (CME) based on the small group learning format. This method of adult learning, led by a suitably rained CME tutor, has been highly successful and indeed has been copied by many similar groups around the world. This is not to say that lectures and demonstrations by hospital consultants are never used as part of CME today, but the pre-eminence of the value of the GP tutor-led small groups has awakened the general practitioners to the key active role *they* can play in keeping themselves up to date.

While the content of the small group meetings is determined by the learners themselves, it is the process that is equally, if not more, important. Instead of being lectured at, these adult learners share their experiences of day-to-day practice problems and use the literature, including valuable guidelines and protocols published by the Irish College of General Practitioners and others, to enable them to improve the standard of their work with patients. In addition, group members can videotape themselves in consultation with selected patients and can then study their consultation behaviour with a view to improving their communication skills. With the decrease in paternalism in today's medical practice and the increasing recognition of the importance of counselling as distinct from advising patients, today's family doctors in training are seeking more counselling skills in an effort to enable patients to help themselves through behavioural change. In the area of loss alone, where doctors in the past might have been tempted to prescribe a mild tranquilliser or anti-depressant for a grief-stricken patient, it is now more common to see such doctors put aside their prescription pads in favour of giving the patient more time, higher quality listening and an emphasis on the innate strengths and resources of the individual to cope with his or her psychological pain, as part of a vital process of personal growth and development. Such adult learning is also leading to doctors themselves developing insights into their own behaviour and mental health needs. Historically, it was always assumed that doctors were strong, healthy people who were programmed to survive all manner of external attack, including bacteria, viruses and the stresses of their daily work. Today, however, doctors have come to realise the importance of recognising their own vulnerabilities and the need to take better care of themselves before attempting to take care of others. It is now recognised that doctors can also become patients and therefore need to 'practise what they preach' by ensuring balance in their personal lives. It has been a tradition in medicine to 'grin and bear it' and not to show one's own feelings and vulnerabilities in case one might be judged 'unfit for office'. In the postgraduate vocational training programme at the Royal College of Surgeons in Ireland, the young doctors in training for general practice greatly value their module on 'personal and professional growth' which is facilitated by a psychotherapist. Here, in the safe and intimate setting of the small group, trainees are encouraged to share their feelings, including their fears, about becoming a general practitioner and the importance of seeking support when it is needed. Although, initially quite threatening to young doctors who have been raised in another culture – the competitive environment of the medical school – it soon becomes clear to all involved that the opposite to sharing and supporting is often denial and isolation, which ultimately can lead to depression, alcohol or drug abuse, and even suicide in up to 10 per cent of doctors who ultimately can no longer cope.

Attention is rightly given to the importance of continuous professional development for general practitioners. Emphasis is placed on their keeping up with moving points in medicine such as information technology, evidence-based medicine, practice organisation and management team development, acquisition of new skills such as counselling, and the role of palliative medicine in the setting of general practice. The new discipline of evidence-based medicine has now been formalised into a major subject in medical education today. While the discipline of evidence-based medicine is of value to the family doctor, it is often the case that there is little or no evidence in the medical literature to guide him or her in many clinical and non-clinical decisions. With the rise in the interest in clinical audit, however, general practitioners will themselves identify areas of their daily work which is based on flimsy or no evidence and be prompted to carry out their own research. This, in turn, may help to provide the evidence that has been lacking in the past. Such lifelong learning, based on insights gleaned from one's own work, represents the very essence of keeping up-to-date and is to be nurtured and invested in, so that tomorrow's doctors will first, be more rounded, mature human beings and secondly, be capable of identifying their own ongoing learning needs. This should lead them to devise ways and means of addressing their needs from a combination of their own resources as well as those from a wide range of other disciplines, including hospital specialists, non-medical carers such as psychologists and social workers, community based nurses, practice managers and information technology personnel such as medical librarians.

Role of other professionals in maximising Irish general practice

While the cornerstone of Irish general practice is still the single-handed family doctor working largely on his or her own, significant inputs are now being made to the discipline by a variety of health-related personnel. Chief amongst these in recent times has been the practice nurse who, together with the general practitioner and practice receptionist/secretary, often forms the core team for provision of care to a practice population of about two thousand people. Other personnel who may work closely with general practice are the public health nurse, a counsellor or psychotherapist and a practice manager, especially for a group practice.

The practice nurse

It has only been in the past decade or so that nurses have moved from largely hospital-based practice to work in the community, specifically in the general practice setting. Here the practice nurse makes a significant contribution to patient care. In the first instance, the practice nurse supports the general practitioner in the first-line care of acutely ill patients, such as the person in an asthmatic attack. Secondly, she monitors patients with chronic or long-term illness attending the practice. Thirdly, she takes the initiative in preventative medicine programmes, such as immunisation and cervical smears. Finally, she is the key educator of patients, always reminding people that they alone can modify their unhealthy lifestyles and take responsibility for their own health. She is thus a major player on the modern general practice primary care team.

The public health nurse

In 2004 there were approximately 3,000 public health nurses attached to and employed by the community care departments of health boards throughout the country. They were supervised by a superintendent public health nurse for each health board and worked from the administrative headquarters of the employing authority.[1] Public health nurses receive their workload in a variety of ways, including referral of discharged patients from hospital and referrals from general practitioners. In addition to their acute and chronic patient workload, they are also responsible for visiting the housebound and elderly in their own homes, as well as visiting mothers and their young babies recently discharged from maternity hospitals to ensure that all is well in the post-natal period and that the baby will be registered for primary immunisation, normally with their family doctor. The public health nurse has an important role in preventive medicine, including the recognition of early developmental problems in the

1   Editor's note. In 2003 the government announced proposals for the abolition of the health boards (see McCluskey, chapter 14).

infant or young child and encouragement of breast-feeding, wherever possible. She has a very varied role which includes the compilation of an at-risk register for her community care team as well as the reporting of any child at risk to the relevant authorities.

The counsellor or psychotherapist

It is only in very recent times that family doctors have come to appreciate the valuable contribution which a counsellor or psychotherapist can make to a practice. This contribution is at least twofold. First, the counsellor or psycho-therapist can see clients directly or on referral for assessment and counselling where appropriate. Patients who are particularly suited are those who are going through a life crisis, have suffered the loss of a loved one or are suffering from anxiety and depression precipitated by a host of possible causes or events. Second, the counsellor or psychotherapist has a valuable role in educating the doctors and other members of the primary care team about the various options available to their patients other than those provided along traditional medical lines, such as prescribing medication or referral to a psychiatrist. The Irish College of General Practitioners has published a comprehensive document on this aspect of general practice as doctors have grown to appreciate both the limitations of medicine and the innate power of their patients to heal themselves, given expert psychological guidance and support (O'Carroll and O'Riordan, 1996).

The practice manager

Most practices are run or managed by the single-handed doctor or, in the case of a group, by consensus of the partners. In more recent times, doctors have come to appreciate the value of employing a suitably trained professional person to manage the practice overall, so as to enable them to focus their time and energies on their clinical work. Some of the advantages of employing a practice manager include: utilising resources to maximum efficiency; managing change in the practice; managing the practice finances; ensuring an appropriate skills mix in the practice and a planned response to patient needs; developing the practice team through the imaginative use of 'away-days' and team-building exercises; preparing and helping to implement a business plan in consultation with the practice partners; employing staff and engaging in regular staff appraisals towards continuous staff development.

While group practices of three or more partners are still in the minority in Ireland, it is increasingly likely that smaller practices will combine to engage a manager on a part-time or shared basis, in order to achieve the benefits outlined above. Already there are several examples of shared management in the UK, sometimes with as many as three practices sharing the one manager.

Retrospect and prospect

In the early years of the twenty-first century, it is timely to reflect on where we have come from and where we are going at this time of significant change in Irish general practice. The family doctor or general practitioner as we know him or her arose from the dispensary doctor service which began in the latter half of the nineteenth century and continued largely unchanged up to the inception of the General Medical Service scheme in 1970. The General Medical Service scheme (GMS) is also known as the Choice of Doctor Scheme, which at its foundation was an important reference to the fact that patients who were eligible for free GMS services had free choice of doctor, at least within a seven-mile radius of their homes. Today, GMS eligible patients still have that right to choose, which extends to having the right to change doctors if patients wish to do so. This underlying principle of freedom of choice was and is deemed important in order to give GMS eligible patients the same right of choice which is automatically available to the private, fee-paying patient. There is also an important choice of patient clause in the GMS contract whereby a general practitioner may request the removal of a patient from his or her list by the health board, should the doctor/patient relationship break down irretrievably. Irish general practice has made considerable strides towards better services for patients, especially since the inception of the GMS scheme in 1970. First amongst these, perhaps, was the establishment of the Irish College of General Practitioners in 1984.

Looking to the future it is never easy to predict how a particular discipline or branch of a profession may develop. In the 1960s it was fashionable for surgeons to frown upon keyhole surgery, while day-case surgery was confined to minor procedures such as circumcision of children or the removal of toenails and simple cysts. Today, thirty years on, the world of day-case surgery has changed beyond recognition. In many cases, established surgeons have had to undergo considerable retraining in order to develop new skills in minimally invasive surgery such as the use of the laparoscope and the arthroscope, as well as to develop highly technical skills in laser surgery. In the case of general practice, I predict a number of significant changes in improving patient care. The following is perhaps more by way of a personal wish list than any accurate emissions from gazing into the fallible crystal ball! Some of the developments I would like to see include the following:

- An increasing role for family doctors in the education of all medical students, who might study more about health in the future and less about the minutiae of disease.
- An expanded postgraduate training curriculum from three to four years, so as to better equip tomorrow's family doctors to deal with patients

and families troubled more by psychological problems than by traditional diseases.

- Planned opportunities for the retraining of family doctors in new skills and special interests such as palliative care in the home and the use of information technology, to name but two; this could be achieved by the imaginative use of sabbatical leave for family doctors who rarely, if ever, enjoy this particular luxury.
- The establishment of a system of patient registration for all citizens in Ireland both for the GMS and private patients, so as to maximise the potential in general practice for preventive medicine and patient education, which is currently not often taken up by patients in the private sector. The current 'non-system' whereby private or fee-paying patients may visit any one of a number of family doctors is unsatisfactory and leads to poor record keeping and tracing of patients for recall for preventive procedures such as immunisation and cervical smears, to name but two.
- The amalgamation of single-handed and two-person practices wherever possible into more viable groups and teams so as to maximise the potential for the better use of resources and the provision of a wider range of services to patients and clients.
- The transfer of more resources from secondary to primary care in parallel with the transfer of an increasing number of patients from the secondary to the primary sector, such as the discharge of patients who have been under long-term psychiatric care into the community. The transfer of resources, including personnel and finance, in this manner would also enable patients to have certain diagnostic procedures and minor operations carried out in the family doctor's surgery, rather than in the hospital.
- The appointment of more managers in general practice either in a large group practice or shared between smaller practices so as to maximise resources, while facilitating team development and the implementation of agreed changes for better patient care.
- The involvement of registered patients in a practice in decision making about the range and quality of services to be provided by the primary care team, including the family doctor.
- The placement of trainees from other health care disciplines in suitably selected training practices so as to broaden their understanding of the setting of primary care. I see this as being particularly relevant and valuable for hospital doctors training in specialties closely related to family medicine, such as paediatrics, care of the elderly and psychiatry. Such attachments might also be usefully extended to trainee counsellors or psychotherapists, nurses and social workers.
- The development of a network of research practices, so as to involve them in research studies of relevance to patients in the community.

Chapter 10

Patient roles, present and future

Tony O'Sullivan

It is a reasonable statement that health policy development in Ireland has been modelled on the middle ground between British and American models. Many would say we have been striving for American heights, but with British resources. In one respect, however, we have fallen well behind both countries. That is in the area of patient rights and responsiveness to the consumer.

In Britain, these rights are supported by a local network of independent watchdogs with funding and statutory rights. These community health councils are formed from the community, and are both accessible and transparent in their actions. In a recent National Health Service (NHS) review, these have been replaced by the more comprehensive Patient Advocacy and Liaison Service (PALS). In the United States, patient rights are largely protected through civil court actions, and while many of the consequences of this have been beneficial (for example, an increased emphasis on adequate consent and full discussions of proposed treatment), many are destructive, including the high rates of 'negative' defensive practices such as caesarean section, the withdrawal of services completely from many communities, and substantial inequality in access to health care fuelled by the high costs of medical indemnity and unnecessary tests and treatments performed 'just in case'.

Ireland has escaped much of this change, and many physicians returning from abroad are surprised at the persistence of paternalistic models of the doctor–patient relationship. This model was the norm throughout the twentieth century, and older patients are often confused and surprised by requests to make decisions about their care, having never needed to do this before.

What's wrong with paternalism?

Paternalism implies a power relationship between doctor – or nurse, administrator or any other health care functionary – and patient which leaves the patient at a distinct disadvantage. On the face of it, there would be little wrong with a trusted medical expert making a balanced judgement about what course of action might be in the patient's best interests. Nevertheless, there are difficulties with this for an increasing majority of patients and doctors. In particular, the doctor cannot make a complete judgement without an in-depth understanding of the patient's value structures, and this is not usually attainable in a short relationship such as during hospitalisation for an acute illness.

For example, a patient may have a fear of surgery driven by the experiences of a relative or friend, but have no such concern about radiotherapy. When faced with prostate cancer, his specialist may have the opposite view and conclude that surgery is the best option. He may wish to spare the patient from having to make a difficult choice by only discussing surgery with him, even though either would be equally effective. Terrified, the patient defaults from all treatment and says he would rather let nature take its course.

Further, the environment of paternalism does not lend itself to differing from the doctor's point of view, or clarifying areas of concern. Paternalism implies a difference in status between doctor and patient which can be misrepresented. Certainly, the doctor is highly qualified, comfortable in the health care environment, possesses the language of the expert, and is treated with deference by other staff, but as a consequence he often overestimates his own status, and thus underestimates that of the patient.

In addition, paternalism assumes roles well beyond the area of clarifying difficult medical choices into regions which are unrelated to the doctor's expertise and exceed his area of influence. This area permits individual professionals to wield sometimes enormous power and hold unassailable positions, and is clearly open to abuse in the context of inadequate regulation. Since 1997, Patient Focus and its predecessor, the Irish Patients Association, have responded to hundreds of stories ranging from misunderstanding to coercion, from rejection on economic grounds to treatment without consent, from discourtesy to assault and sexual abuse. Not all of these experiences are the direct consequence of paternalism, but many stem from a continuing acceptance of this model.

Patients in difficulty

Over the years, Patient Focus has built up a picture of how deeply people are affected by negative health care experiences. Patient Focus has also seen the therapeutic effects many have obtained from simply describing these experiences, even by letter to a distant but supportive stranger. For most people, their needs are not unachievable; indeed, they are surprisingly simple. Even after losing a spouse or child, most of the correspondents ask only for an explanation or apology, and for assurances that an avoidable tragedy will not be repeated.

An attempt has been made to assess the frequency of these problems, as it is suspected that of the thousand or more contacts made to Patient Focus, these may be only the tip of the iceberg. On behalf of Patient Focus, Lansdowne Market Research conducted a national survey of a representative sample of adults in June/July 1999, asking 1,400 respondents aged 15 or over about hospital attendance during the previous five years. A total of 643 respondents (46%) recalled attending hospital as either inpatients or outpatients over that period. Those attending were asked a series of questions relevant to patient involvement in decisions, rights issues and satisfaction (table 10.1).

Table 10.1 **Patients' responses to questions relating to their hospital experience**

Question	Percentage responding 'no'	
	Inpatients	Outpatients
Did medical staff introduce themselves?	15	35
Were you fully informed about your condition?	9	17
Was treatment explained in a way you could understand?	9	15
Did nursing staff seem interested in helping you?	5	14
Did all examinations take place in private?	6	10
Were you treated with respect and dignity throughout?	6	8
Percentage rating care as 'bad' or 'terrible' overall	4	8
N	**431**	**174**

Source: Irish Patients' Association and Lansdowne Market Research (1999)

The results confirm that a significant minority of patients were exposed to unacceptable lapses in ordinary standards of care. These lapses seem to be more common in public hospital care than in private, and in outpatient rather than inpatient settings. The results may underestimate difficulties, as surveys frequently overestimate satisfaction, and between three and 15 per cent of respondents answered 'don't know' to specific questions.

Identifying the causes

It has always been the aim of Patient Focus to identify and correct the underlying causes of patients' difficulties, and to do this an open-minded view of where these causes lie is required. An understanding of this area from a patient's perspective has been developed, and the problems identified arise in the following areas: (1) status of the patient; (2) status of the professional; (3) health care environment; (4) health infrastructure.

Status of the patient

For myself and my family our story was and still is a nightmare. We loved my father. He died from septic shock brought on by an infection he got following an ERCP (an investigation based on endoscopy) done ten days previously. I understand anyone can pick up an infection but they usually recover. I suppose his resistance was very low. We visited three times a day. Hounded doctors and nurses for information and got none. My complaint is of their lack of compassion and basic human kindness. We wrote down our phone number for the nurse, put it in her pocket, to save her having to look it up if his condition deteriorated during the night. Little did we know of the events of the night. In these situations you tend to think no news is good news. We were told by other patients of the bad night he had. One patient held his hand and tried to calm him and I am so grateful to him for that but I am miserable that it wasn't my mother. Surely 46 years of marriage warrants that special privilege. It was barbaric that they never rang. Patients are just an object . . . The fact that they are somebody's husband or father is of no consequence to them. I enclose a photo to remind you that it is a human being not a patient or a file number that I write to you about. (A daughter describing her father's death)

Few Irish people have a clear understanding of their rights as patients. That these rights will be protected is assumed, although many are sorely disappointed. Rights are often denied without a patient or his family being fully aware that this is the case. Patient Focus learned of an elderly man residing as a long-stay patient in a state institution. His family called one Saturday to take him out for the day and were told he was not allowed to go, as punishment for some behavioural misdemeanour. Initially, they had accepted this, even though such restraint is plainly illegal.

Similarly, many patients give accounts of unacceptable practices, from the use of restraints to tie people to chairs or beds, to major surgery without consent, and yet they are uncertain about whether or not the practice really is wrong. This uncertainty is a clear barrier to the correction of deficiencies in the system. Further, many patients and relatives approach Patient Focus with feelings of resignation about events, believing that there is little or no accountability for wrongdoing.

Clearly, patients need and deserve to be informed about their rights at the time they become involved with health care. They also need local, independent protection of those rights, and this cannot be achieved without the creation of a fully-funded, locally-based service along similar lines to the PALS in the UK. Roles for such a service would include public education, starting at school, about how to use health services effectively, and what rights those using services in Ireland can expect to enjoy; providing an overview of safe and effective care, managing a statutory complaints services and advising the Minister and those responsible for professional training and regulation.

The status of vulnerable patients is particularly difficult. These groups are open to substantial abuse, and it is reasonable to suppose that this vulnerability in some way reflects the status of those groups in Irish society. Health simply mirrors the social attitudes of the nation. Advocates have always been concerned for the protection of older people and children, and those with handicap or mental illness, for example, but asylum seekers, members of the Travelling community, and prisoner and other groups present new challenges. The range of eligibility for services does not improve matters, adding a financial disincentive to providing safe care to poorly remunerated groups. There is adequate evidence of the different treatment of some patients with medical cards, for example. Surprisingly, private health care presents its own problems, ranging from a reduced level of contact with medical or nursing personnel, to a lack of supporting medical services when things go wrong.

Status of the professional

I am still annoyed with myself when I remember that I didn't have the courage to complain about the behaviour of two consultants, one of whom regularly tore open the buttons of elderly ladies' nighties during ward rounds without warning them or excusing himself and the other who demonstrated how to take the pulse at the top of the leg by shoving his hand up their nighties, again without asking permission. (A young woman doctor talking about her recent medical student days)

Medical education produces doctors with superb clinical skills, but who are poorly prepared for working in teams with professional colleagues or in partnership with patients. One of the things doctors learn is that communicating with patients is less valuable than using clinical skills or investigations, and such communication is the first area to suffer under the pressure of long hours and severe workloads. Detailed explanations are an unnecessary chore to many doctors, and many patients and relatives have told us that doctors refused to meet or discuss cases with them, even after serious mishaps or the unexpected death of a patient. Much patient communication is delegated to junior staff who are not equipped for the task. It is a matter of routine in most hospitals that one of the regular tasks for the intern – the most junior grade of doctor – is to obtain patients' consent. This is a problem when the doctor does not know enough about the patient's condition, the planned treatment, its side effects or the alternatives. There are many instances of patients giving uncertain consent to uncertain doctors relating to difficult, marginal treatment decisions with life-or-death implications.

Doctors are often described as arrogant by patients, and communication problems contribute to this, not only in the apparent refusal to communicate, but in the deliberate use of medical jargon. These traits are in evidence at all levels in the profession, so their correction requires action at established as well as at training grades. Current changes in undergraduate medical education include earlier contact with patients and a gradual erosion of pre-clinical basic sciences in favour of training in the skills and attitudes of communication, disease management, ethical deliberation and self-initiated learning. Patient Focus would like to see awareness training of the needs of different patient groups, shared training with other medical professionals, and professional conflict resolution included with these changes.

This emphasis on establishing effective communication must continue during higher professional training, and should become a part of continuing professional development (CPD) for established doctors and other professionals. The Medical Council has recently proposed a system of competence assurance. In essence, all established doctors would be obliged to complete a number of tasks, including CPD, peer review and clinical audit, to maintain their name on the register of medical practitioners. This is to be applauded as a protection against a minority of professionals who make little or no effort to keep up with current standards or practices, and who can become harmful to patients as a result. Moreover, this system would also create an opportunity to give communication skills and related issues a deserved educational priority.

Training is only one of many aspects of professional development. Peer review has long been accepted by many specialists as an effective exercise in standardising the level of care provided to patients across the country. This is supplemented by local guidelines and standards. While guidelines have limitations they are a protection against the potential excesses of 'clinical freedom'. This point remains a source of potential conflict between the profession, on the one hand, and patients, insurers and employers on the other, particularly since clinical autonomy is written into the existing consultants' contract. Whatever its eventual format, CPD and competence assurance activities will need to be encouraged by those who pay for health, including health authorities, employers and health insurers. It should further attract benefits including reduced indemnity premiums as occur in the USA.

Health care environment

As I write I can still feel the anger rising at how my mother and I were treated. It was a litany of bad manners. To be questioned, was it seems a downright slap in the face [to consultants] and we felt we really were for it after we had the nerve to question the way we were treated. I could write a book about it. I hope you can feel the depth of hatred we now have for the medical system. (A nurse writing about her mother's cancer treatment)

The employment environment in Irish health care has never been conducive to protecting the interests of patients. Factors inhibiting the investigation of an employee's concerns about a colleague include the lack of any administrative arrangements for listening to such concerns, and a lack of protection for a whistle-blowing staff member. For instance, doctors have admitted that these concerns have led to them to protecting a surgeon with an alcohol problem, despite the risk to patients.

Many ongoing tragedies would have been curtailed if patients had a *safe* conduit for their views and concerns. Few patients feel they will be heard if they raise a concern. We have established that few Irish health institutions have an adequate protocol for receiving and handling the concerns of patients or their families, and almost none have a policy which *encourages* such views. A fundamental feature of health care risk-management is just such encouragement. Many tragedies may be prevented by encouraging patients' views. When professionals feel inhibited from expressing concerns, or simply do not notice problems, patients can be a useful resource indeed.

Of course, patients can also feel inhibited from making their views known. The vocational nature of Irish health care engenders a feeling amongst providers that they are beyond reproach. Staff have been slighted by even the most ordinary questioning of their expertise. Patients fear that their care, or that of their loved one, will suffer if they complain. In the experience of Patient Focus, such fears may not be unfounded. One group of patients attending a unit in a major hospital met as a group, discussed common problems relating to their care in the unit, and came up with proposals for correcting a number of these problems. When they presented these proposals to those in charge of the unit, they were side-lined by an unimpressive display of inter-professional mistrust, churlish ill feeling amongst the staff, and several episodes of ill treatment of the patients involved.

Among the solutions to this problem are initiatives such as the identification of a patient services officer or, better, an adequate complaints procedure, including regular feedback to the complainant and prompt, satisfactory resolution including instituting changes where appropriate. In the experience of Patient Focus, patients who complain about their care are seeking very modest, achievable aims, including an apology and some sign that efforts will be made to prevent the same thing happening to someone else. It is unfortunate then that much of the response to complaints ignores these needs, and focuses instead on preventing the patient from taking a civil action. A number of people have said that they were driven to seeing a solicitor, and hence to litigation, by the refusal of an institution to respond to basic requests for information.

The private hospital sector is a particular cause for concern. Care is provided almost exclusively by the patient's consultant, supported by a small medical staff employed by the hospital. There is essentially no consultant accountability in this sector as the doctor is not an employee. Administrators in this sector have told me that they cannot afford to uphold a patient's complaint against a consultant as they rely on consultants to bring patients to the hospital. In this tense symbiosis the protection of patients' interests is clearly secondary.

It is no longer acceptable that patients are denied opportunities to participate in the planning of health services, locally or nationally. Failing to involve patients produces services that are bereft of their valuable advice and insensitive to their needs. The approach of coroners and pathologists in children's hospitals to post-mortem examinations on deceased children has been criticised as seriously insensitive by many parents, and for some constitutes a violation of their dead children.

On a more positive note, St Joseph's Hospital in Clonmel has developed an innovative and possibly unique patient user group. The group meets regularly along with senior nursing and administrative staff, and when this writer arrived to attend one meeting they were discussing plans for a multi-million pound extension to the hospital with its architect. The patients made sensible and valuable comments which can only enhance the planning of such expenditure on their behalf.

For patient groups to work, they must be truly representative of the population served, and have genuine influence at the most senior level in the institution. The Voluntary Health Insurance (VHI) Board has a user group which is entirely convened from large employee group schemes, and in the past this group has criticised the company for failing to respond to its reports. Most health boards and authorities were dominated by political and professional members, with public interest representatives heavily outnumbered. In recent years, health boards had sought a wider input from the public into the medium-term planning of services. Through a combination of their own inexperience and the public's lengthy experience of being ignored, it was difficult for them to obtain a satisfactory response to their calls for submissions.

Patient Focus has long campaigned for increased patient involvement at all levels in the health services. Carefully prepared focus groups have contributed to difficult decisions about the distribution of funds in the UK and elsewhere, even to the extent of agreeing to hospital closures – which politicians find unacceptably difficult to do on their own. Patient Focus believes that the established role of carers and the voluntary sector remains unacknowledged and utterly unrewarded in Ireland. Health care administrators take the continued goodwill of these groups for granted at their peril. There are signs of escalating discontent with the hardship of the caring lifestyle, and the cost to the state of a large-scale rejection of home care for the elderly would be enormous. Such change has occurred in the UK, and will follow here, if the plight of carers continues to be ignored.

Health care infrastructure

Change requires resources and political support, but in Ireland politics has an uneasy relationship with health care. It is a cumbersome ministry, fraught with industrial relations problems and with competing claims on resources, most of them very desirable and valid. Services appear to evolve in a disjointed and inequitable way. Currently, one would get the impression that many decisions are taken in an ad hoc way, and in some cases are frankly misguided. Representatives of the huge, youthful local catchment area remain confused at the failure to provide a maternity unit at Tallaght Hospital. The abrupt withdrawal of services from the south inner city left many patients struggling with inadequate public transport services to Tallaght. The ensuing transfer of many city-dwelling patients to St James's, and the corresponding transfer of people from Dublin 24 to the Tallaght site, should have been predicted and planned for. Meanwhile, the closure of the National Children's Hospital in Harcourt Street has left the south-east of Dublin with no paediatric service.

Dublin's problems aside, the provision of services to the remainder of the country is at best patchy, at worst waiting in hopeful expectation. Successive governments have pledged to overcome health care inequity, yet cancer patients from Donegal have to travel to Dublin (and find accommodation at their own expense) for radiotherapy treatment despite being at their most vulnerable following surgery or chemotherapy and needing the support of their families more than ever. Despite numerous reports and strategies, the regional distribution of specialist services such as cancer treatment is still undeveloped.

A child falling and cutting his or her face will have access to specialist plastic surgery care, but only if they live in Dublin, Cork or Galway. Everywhere else she will be patched up by the GP, a casualty officer or surgeon. If she has a serious head injury she had better be in Dublin or Cork. The health service is rife with specialties available in several sites in Dublin, and nowhere else. One solution to such centralisation is a well-resourced ambulance service. In fact, the ambulance services are seriously inadequate, and there is no helicopter ambulance for major accidents or the transfer of seriously ill patients across the country.

There is also much economic inequality in Irish health services. Many people just outside the income limit for the medical card suffer restricted access to preventive care as a result and it is a barrier to the effective transfer of care for conditions such as diabetes and minor injuries from hospital to general practice. The public hospital service has a number of co-payments – such as a fee for casualty attendance and a daily charge for inpatient treatment – which act as a disincentive to the less well-off to make any use of services, appropriate or otherwise. VHI members get this money back, and medical cardholders don't pay it, but those who are just ineligible for a medical card, and their children, pay in full. Those without a medical card also have to pay a substantial amount each month for medication. People with some conditions such as diabetes can obtain their medicines free on a 'long-term illness' scheme, but those with asthma cannot. Such barriers are essentially a crude form of rationing, and they discriminate on economic grounds rather than providing services on the basis of need.

Health Strategy, 2001

The Health Strategy 2001 comprises two documents. The first, *Quality and Fairness, a Health System for You* (Department of Health and Children, 2001a) specifies a series of essential actions to achieve the goals of the Strategy. An accompanying document *Primary Care: A New Direction* (Department of Health and Children, 2001b) sets out details of the new model of primary care contained in the Strategy. The Strategy was influenced by a large consultative forum of over a hundred people from all aspects of health care, and by submissions invited from organisations and individuals. Submissions were received from over 1,500 individuals and 300 organisations.

The consultative forum had a noticeable weighting in favour of patient groups and their representatives. Much work was completed in a very short time, and the resulting documents are an excellent demonstration of the value of public participation in health planning (Department of Health and Children, 2001c). For example, the basic themes for the Strategy were defined in terms of equality, people-centredness, quality and accountability.

A total of 141 specific actions are specified in the Strategy's two documents, covering a broad range of patient groups (from older people to the Travelling community), conditions (mental health, paediatrics, renal and transplant services and progress on existing cancer and healthy heart strategies) and structures (3,000 new hospital beds by 2011, several new authorities). People-centredness is covered by commitments to better health information, a renewed interest in patient satisfaction, integrated care planning to involve patients, and consumer panels and other measures to involve patients in local health care planning.

Quality care is to be managed by a new health information and quality agency. The main strands will be risk management systems and the implementation of protocols and standards in many areas. Transfusion medicine, an area fraught with scandal and tragedy since 1990, receives a special mention. In addition to preventing tragedies, the new emphasis on quality will serve two other important functions: improvement in cost-effectiveness, and opportunities to make professionals more accountable.

Accountability has been used in its most negative context in Irish health care, and this emphasis continues in the Strategy. It revolves around new regulations for doctors, nurses and other health professions, legislation to control alternative practitioners and their therapies, and an enhanced role for the Ombudsman along with a statutory complaints process. These measures are important, but the opportunity for more positive accountability seems to have been missed.

The most obvious gap in the Strategy is a reform in health service funding. Another distinct disappointment was the lack of commitment to remove eligibility discrimination from primary care. An extension of the medical card scheme to the entire population would certainly have offered more equity than any other initiative, and would have enabled the aspirations of the primary care strategy to be realised.

Patient focus

> I should be very grateful if you could advise me as to the course I should take in order to get a full explanation of my brother's treatment . . . and also advise should doctors treat members of the public with contempt and rudeness at a time of distress? I should stress that it is not our intention to seek any financial compensation, we just want to know the full facts surrounding my brother's illness, treatment and death. My brother went into hospital a healthy man to have investigations for gallstones and died 6 weeks later. (A sister seeking advice as to how to get an explanation for her brother's death)

As a national body representing all patients, including future patients, and their families, Patient Focus is unique. Many groups of current patients are represented by disease support groups, like the Irish Heart Foundation or the Cancer Society. Similarly, in the past, individual patients have sought representation from their TD, the Ombudsman, or the Minister for Health and Children. Unlike all of these, Patient Focus is independent of the professions, institutions and the administration; it is open to everybody regardless of diagnosis or if there is no diagnosis; it does not require membership or request payment of any kind from patients, and crucially it offers *unquestioning* support, so that patients know that we are always going to side with them. This last is not the risk that it may sound, and is the only effective way to obtain the trust of patients who have often suffered a terrible betrayal of trust.

When faced with a patient in serious difficulty, Patient Focus becomes involved at their pace and only acts with their approval. It aims to achieve resolution of the problem as the patient sees it, using available services where possible. This might simply involve encouraging a patient's general practitioner to obtain a second opinion, helping somebody to obtain copies of their medical record, obtaining an apology, improvement in a service or simply an explanation of events. Occasionally it involves attending court proceedings with a patient, or contacting the Gardaí on their behalf. Patients have approached Patient Focus with problems while still in hospital, and about events dating back to the 1940s. Unresolved experiences do not fade, so active resolution even of long-past events is felt to be worth the trouble by the majority of our clients.

Litigation is perceived as a social disease in Ireland, yet it should be unnecessary if people harmed by health care were offered reasonable compensation. Patient Focus do not encourage civil actions, nor does it discourage them, since many people view them as a suitable form of justice. Patient Focus hopes to develop alternative means of settling health care disputes, which may prove acceptable to frustrated patients and providers alike. Mediation is a proven mechanism for the early resolution of patients' concerns, and offers real explanations, apologies and modest compensation where appropriate. The format is conciliatory rather than adversarial, and the two sides are represented by a minimum of legal personnel, making it very cost-effective for either side.

Patient Focus also acts to adjust the system in patients' favour, through professional education, political discussion, interaction with providers and professional groups and through publishing occasional reports. Previous projects include discussions with the Medical Council, the Ombudsman and political leaders, participation in conferences and quality development projects, research into hospital complaints procedures, and preparing invited submissions for government. Recent projects have included negotiation with health boards on the development of consumer panels; continuing involvement in new Medical Council procedures, participation in the Commission on Child Abuse and continuing to seek support for a fully developed patient advocacy service.

Part 4

Disability issues

Chapter 11

The contours of learning/ intellectual disability

Máiríde Woods

This chapter is written from the perspective of a parent who is a writer, sociologist and researcher, an intermittent campaigner on disability matters and a member of the board of a voluntary organisation. One of my daughters had Rett Syndrome, which causes multiple disabilities). I use the following definition of intellectual/learning disability, accepted by the World Health Organisation (WHO), which describes people with intellectual disabilities as having:

> significantly sub-average general intellectual functioning existing concurrently with deficits in adaptive behaviour and manifested during the development period. (http://www.ucaqld.com.au/disability/id.html)

How does learning disability fit into a book about health policy and practice in Ireland? Does it belong at all? The fact that this essay begins with such questions signals how much has changed in concepts and attitudes concerning learning disability in Ireland of today.

So why consider learning disability in the context of health? After all, it is restrictive to locate disability there. The crude answer is that the Department of Health and Children is the major source of both policy and funding for Irish learning disability services. It is therefore necessary to maintain a profile with that department and to disseminate changing values and attitudes to the policy makers. There is limited usefulness in disabled people preaching the social model to each other, while the professionals and Department of Health and Children officials continue in the medical model of their training. And while people with mild or moderate learning disability may have little need to interact with the medical profession, this is not the case for those with severe or profound learning disability. Both families and the medical profession need to understand and influence the other's positions and concerns.

Terminology

I use the term 'learning disability' because it is the one most widely acceptable at present. The Disability Movement has rejected the term 'handicap' as being resonant of the old approach to disability – the person as object of pity; and a similar attitude has been taken to 'mental handicap'. Some people with mild learning disability also feel that the 'mental' sobriquet suggests mental illness. Labelling theory – the idea that a label like mental handicap evokes stereotyped expectations and responses – has also been influential.

Changes in language can cause difficulties. The Department of Health and Children uses the term 'intellectual disability' (Guidon, 1990), which has been slow to gain general acceptance in Ireland although the organisation NAMHI (formerly National Association of People with Mental Handicap in Ireland) has included 'People with intellectual disabilities' in its new name. The fluidity of the terms 'learning disability' and 'learning difficulties' can lead to misunderstanding. Learning disability is also used for conditions such as dyslexia. 'Learning difficulties' or 'delayed development' can devalue the extent of the problem to parents and teachers. These terms may reflect a reluctance by doctors and psychologists to give an exact medical assessment to the parent of the child with a learning disability. Switching labels can help change people's attitudes, but may also suggest that the disability has vanished, and no services or supports are needed. If other changes are not made new labels will take on the old connotations. Some evaluation is inevitable in assessment and in devising appropriate services. To keep the assessment criteria hidden in order to avoid controversy or offence does not respect the person or their family. An exact label can help understanding of the person's potential and limitations. When my own daughter's condition finally received a name (when she was 15), I was on the whole relieved as it gave us an explanation and parameters.

Changes in the construction and understanding of learning disability

The disability movement both in Ireland and abroad has put a salutary question mark over what used to be considered natural in the field of disability. This questioning of the natural and the taken-for-granted is part of many postmodernist interpretations of the social world. It used to appear natural to associate disability with medicine and rehabilitation, but that was partly a result of the prestige of medicine in the nineteenth and early twentieth centuries (Stone, 1984). Doctors were seen as independent arbiters of disability – both of its genuineness and its extent. Twentieth-century medicine, however, concentrates on cure, and because disability can at best only be managed, it represents a degree of failure to doctors. This may partly explain the earlier trend to segregate disabled people in institutions, although the extreme poverty of many people's living conditions was also a factor.

The medical model of disability emphasised the individual impairment, the departure from the norm, the tragedy for the individual, the need for rehabilitation. In many countries (USA, Germany, Sweden) there was a eugenic strand to this argument which most people today find shocking. Some policy makers saw a possible danger to national health if 'defective' individuals were allowed to reproduce. It is not surprising that this model has been robustly challenged by disabled people who see their cause as the last struggle for civil rights. Their model – the social model – stresses the disabling and oppressive effects of the barriers erected, deliberately or thoughtlessly, by mainstream society (Oliver, 1991). In this view, society has a responsibility to make arrangements and practices as inclusive as possible; where specialist services are needed, these should as far as is practicable be provided, not in special ghettos which can become empires for the professional 'denizens of the disability industry' (Oliver 1991), but in the mainstream – for example within ordinary schools and workplaces. The social model has grown in tandem with a rights-based approach, which sees services as something owed to the person by virtue of citizenship. Its most tangible effect has been the United States Americans with Disabilities Act, which in 1990 outlawed discrimination in employment and services on the grounds of disability. The Irish Employment Equality Act 1998 and the Equal Status Act 2000 drew much of their inspiration from such legislation; many people saw the fact that disability was rubbing shoulders with eight other grounds of possible discrimination as normalising disability and placing the emphasis on the discriminatory acts rather than on special treatment. The influence of the EU (through the Framework directives) and the European Convention on Human Rights have also been positive for disability in Ireland.

One or two cases under the Employment Equality Act have broken some barriers for people with learning disabilities, but it has to be recognised that such legislation sometimes has the unintended effect of making employers wary of taking on anyone who could give rise to a case. This is one of the reasons why education of the public, partnership schemes with employers and a quota system (as envisaged in the Disability Bill 2004) are still needed.

The social model has been empowering for people with disabilities and for their families. Some of its insights have been accepted by the Irish government in its recognition of the philosophy of the Commission on the Status of People with Disabilities (1996), which emphasised the key points of equality, consultation and mainstreaming. There have, however, been setbacks such as the short-lived Disability Bill of 2001 (which fell on the issue of rights) and the snail's pace of physical accessibility. The social model also does not totally fit the learning disability experience. Empowering people with learning disabilities to make the most of their potential can throw up complex problems. Even with optimum conditions, learning disability itself can affect the person's ability to organise his or her life and to make decisions alone. Some 'social model' writers recognise this: 'Although the minority group or social model sometimes seems to argue that all disabilities are social constructs, there are problems related to disability which do not solely arise in a person's environment' (Hendriks, 1995: 59). Treating people with learning disability 'the same' as everyone else (the simplest rights-based approach) may ensure them a precarious existence at the bottom of our social pile – in the lowliest shrink-wrapping jobs. As Martha Minow showed in an article which referred to two famous US cases of the seventies, 'similar treatment' may get people out of the institutions but will not give them the services they need to survive outside (Minow, 1987). The challenge is to find ways of allowing for difference without denying the person's basic human rights. Ensuring flexible, individual and changing levels of supervision and support for people with learning difficulties, while encouraging them to participate in the wider society as far as they can, sets the greatest challenge to providers. For this group, positive discrimination in employment is needed – such as has occurred in some of the supported employment models.

The normalisation approach, pioneered by Wolfensberger (1972), emphasised the similarities between people with learning disability and everyone else, and the need to use an ordinary lifestyle as a yardstick. The slogan has been to concentrate on ability not on disability, and some people with learning disabilities have reached levels of achievement (reading, writing, sport, some Junior Certificate subjects) which would have been unthinkable thirty years ago. But sometimes these very successes can further marginalise those who do not make the hoped-for progress, who have multiple disabilities, or whose behaviour problems persist. Parents sometimes have to square the almost compulsory optimism of the service providers and the disability activists with the realisation that, in the words of the well-known radio reporter, Kevin O'Kelly (1989), 'handicap is hard', and that progress will be measured in terms of very small steps and personal contentment, rather than in conventional achievements.

Numbers of people with learning disability in Ireland

Learning disability in Ireland has the distinction of having over twenty years of reasonably accurate statistics (1981, 1996, 1998, 2000).[1] The health boards used to be responsible for maintaining a database on every individual known to have an intellectual disability or known to be making use of the intellectual disability

---

1   Editor's note. Since the writing of this paper, National Intellectual Disability Database reports have been published for the years 2001 to 2005 inclusive.

services within each health board region. These databases were valuable in validating claims for expanded services and facilitating comprehensive planning; the Equality Authority in its reports has pointed to the need for baseline data to monitor the position of minorities. Any criticisms of the Intellectual Disability Database relate only to methodology and definition, both of which to some extent depend on resources. The collection of readily available information is certainly useful, but full and perfect ascertainment of everyone with any form of learning disability is still some way off.

A National Intellectual Disability Database Report was published by the Health Research Board in 1996, 1998–9 and 2000. In its first report in 1996, it claimed to have achieved almost 100 per cent ascertainment in the areas of moderate, severe and profound intellectual disability. It did not set out its criteria for these divisions, so one assumes they are the traditional ones laid down in the 1981 *Census of Mental Handicap in the Republic of Ireland* (Mulcahy and Reynolds, 1984) and are based on the WHO International Classification of Diseases. In this 1981 census, a psychological assessment was used where possible; otherwise nursing staff made estimates of the person's level of intelligence. The database also relies on reports from the service providers, a method of assessment which could be criticised as variable and not sufficiently searching; it assumes either constant review of people with learning disabilities or a belief that levels of ability do not change. Like the 1981 census, the Database gets over the problem of the cut-off point by counting only those who were either receiving an intellectual disability service, or had applied for, or were likely to need one. Most people with a mild learning disability (general learning difficulties) are probably excluded. This could mean such people do not require a service, or it could mean that the services they need do not exist. The fact that a significant proportion of children who come in contact with the juvenile justice system appear to have general learning difficulties and the setting up of a new group, Borderline, for families of these young people, suggests that mild learning disability can cause considerable problems. Guidon (1990) looked for multi-disciplinary support for this group within the mainstream services.

The chief facts emerging from *The Report on the Intellectual Disability Database* (Health Research Board, 2000) are as follows: there are 26,760 people in Ireland documented as having an intellectual disability, representing a prevalence rate per 1,000 of 7.38. *The Report of the Commission on the Status of People with Disabilities* (Commission, 1996) suggested that people with learning disability make up 10–12 per cent of the estimated total number of disabled people in Ireland. The Census of 2004 put the disabled population at eight per cent.

Forty-one per cent of those on the Intellectual Disability Database (Health Research Board, 2000) fall into the mild category, 36 per cent into the moderate, 15 per cent into the severe, and four per cent into the profound category. The remainder have not been classified. Sixty-one per cent of people live in a home setting, usually with one or both parents. Of those in residential care, almost half are now in community group homes rather than residential centres. However, the most pressing need is still seen to be residential places for adults. The 2000 Report shows that three per cent of all people with learning disability are still in psychiatric hospitals, but it considers that some of these people are 'appropriately placed' (usually because they have a psychiatric disorder).

The 2000 Report (Health Research Board, 2000) shows that 806 (three per cent) of all people with learning disability are still in psychiatric hospitals. This does represent a decrease on the 1996 figure (970) and a considerable decrease on the 1981 figure of 2,321 people resident in such hospitals. The report considers some of these people are 'appropriately placed' (usually because they also have a psychiatric disorder).

Nevertheless, conditions in these hospitals continue to be unsuitable. The Commission on the Status of People with Disabilities (1996) recorded its shock at poor standards of accommodation in one of the psychiatric institutions it visited, and called for a special fund to replace these facilities within five years. But psychiatric hospitals, such as St Ita's in Portrane, County Dublin, still have a mental handicap service within the hospital, and refurbishment is by no means complete.

Both the 1996 and 2000 Reports on the Intellectual Disability Database (Health Research Board, 1996, 2000) highlight the need for geriatric services for some older people with learning disabilities – a consequence of increased life expectancy for people with disability. Down's syndrome is unfortunately correlated with a higher incidence of Alzheimer's disease in middle age. One learning disability service, St Michael's House, took the initiative in 2001 by opening an Alzheimer's unit in north Dublin.

In the area of education, the 2000 Database records 8,307 schoolchildren with learning disabilities, of whom 70 per cent were in special schools or developmental centres, and about 30 per cent in ordinary schools (including special classes). The numbers in day developmental centres (683) have fallen, as, following the O'Donoghue judgment (see below, p. 182), these children are now entitled to a formal education. In the 1981 census 21 per cent of children with learning disability were in ordinary schools; in 1996 the proportion was 25 per cent. Numbers in mainstream schools have not increased as quickly as one would have expected, The National Disability Authority (NDA) research (2001) suggested that not all parents were convinced that mainstream schools could give children with severe disabilities the education they needed. Parents of children with autism have continued to use the judicial review procedure of the courts in their efforts to get appropriate specialised education for their children (Irish Court Reports, 2001).

According to the 2000 Database Report, over 5,000 people with learning disability were in some form of sheltered employment; almost 1,000 were in supported employment and 338 were in open employment. Given the introduction of the Employment Equality Act 1998 and the efforts of agencies and disabled people's groups to promote open employment, the latter figure is disappointing. However, numbers in open employment have trebled since 1996 and the Supported Employment programme – where the employee receives on-the-job back-up – has also seen a major expansion. FÁS (National Employment Training Authority) assumed overall responsibility for training the more able group.

The 1996 and 2000 Database Reports highlight increasing numbers of people with more severe learning disabilities. In spite of the fact that the sharp decline in the birth rate means there are fewer babies with such disabilities, increased life expectancy among people with severe and profound disabilities, coupled with the bulge effect of the numbers born in the late 1960s and early 1970s, account for the increase. This rise has serious implications for services and provision of residential places must continue at the level of 1999 and 2000 if the deficit of earlier years is to be made good. Guidon spoke of the need for 'a clear and certain knowledge on the part of the family that alternative and appropriate accommodation is available . . . immediately it is required' (Guidon, 1990: 9.4). Despite increases in funding and a big expansion in placements between 1999 and 2001, no Irish family that cares for a relative with a learning disability has that certainty.

Move from institutional to community care

Since the 1960s the popularity of institutional care has steadily waned. Originally, community care was seen as providing something human and personalised, without a plethora of rules and regulations. As early as 1965, the Commission of Enquiry on Mental Handicap accepted that care in the community was usually superior to and 'more therapeutic' than institutional care (Department of Health, 1965) and this has been the ideology of services since the 1970s. Community care has cut down on segregation, made disability more visible and familiar, and influenced people with disabilities and their families to demand mainstream standards. It has provided the backdrop for the increased emphasis on equal rights and the move to integration.

The state's espousal of community care may all along have been based on economic factors: it was seen as a less expensive option, because the community boiled down to the family, and the family usually meant the unpaid woman in the home (Finch, 1990). O'Connor (1987) concluded that community care effectively meant family care with little local integration. This will come as little surprise to most parents – my small study reached much the same conclusions (Woods 1997; O'Donoghue-Woods, 1993).

So the costs of disability for people living in their own homes in the community fall disproportionately on them and on their family. Conversely, where a person with severe disability is in residential care, the cost – borne by the state – can be in the region of €30,000 to €50,000 per year. There is thus an inequity between funding for those who live with their families and those who have a residential place. A government committee has been considering a Costs of Disability payment – possibly similar to the UK Disability Living allowance – which would go some way to restoring parity. The fact that in the late 1990s more women in the caring age brackets had opportunities in the paid labour force may have prompted a gradual relaxation of the means test for the carer's allowance. Respite care has also expanded for much the same reason – a fear that the pool of informal carers (mostly women between 45 and 70) could dry up.

'Community care' cornered the rhetoric but not the funding, and the Irish government never spelled out what these words meant. In her 1987 report, Síle O'Connor teased out the blurred meanings of community and care: the former can mean 'setting', 'territory', 'common interests, or 'relationships'; the latter ranges from minimal supervision to total nursing care (O'Connor, 1987). The main misunderstanding seems to be that the state sees community care as chiefly for people without family who would otherwise be in institutions (substitute care); families, on the other hand, often understand community care as the supports they would like in order to care for their disabled member without undue restriction to their own lives (support care).

The community-living model has brought about a considerable improvement in the lifestyle of adults with learning disability. Although the most radical idea was independent living – and this has been possible for a small number of people with learning disabilities – the majority require some type of supervised placement with at least a resident house-parent. Some providers experimented with villages – such as Cheeverstown House in Dublin – where different types of services were provided in small buildings on a large campus-style site, but these have been criticised as too segregated. The more successful option has become small group homes (of about six people) located in ordinary or slightly adapted houses on suburban streets where residents use neighbourhood facilities. Day services also reflect the community approach – many are now located in houses or in school /shop units, each one serving a maximum of about twenty people. The vast majority of children with learning disabilities now live at home with their families.

State supports for people with learning disabilities living in the community include: the Disability Allowance, a means-tested payment for adults; training allowances for people on FÁS courses; the Domiciliary Care Allowance for parents of children with severe disabilities; the Respite Grant; the Mobility

Allowance; the Carer's Allowance; Disabled Person's Housing Grants; and Disabled Driver's and Passenger's Tax Concessions. Most allowances are means-tested and have strict medical condition thresholds as well. When the Carer's Allowance was introduced, the means test (which included a partner's income) meant that few carers qualified. 'Public expenditure on the carer's allowance is very small compared with either (a) opportunity costs to informal carers or (b) the "replacement costs" to public expenditure if care was not provided informally' (Lynch and McLaughlin, 1995). Although adjustments in recent years have allowed more carers to qualify, many are still excluded.

The position of respite care well illustrates how substitute care remains the state's priority. Respite is meant to provide temporary residential care for people with disabilities who live with their families and has expanded in recent years; but where a crisis need for a full-time residential place arises, a respite place is used to fill the gap, thus curtailing the service to parents/ informal carers. The extra funding to cushion a proper change from an institutional system of last resort substitute care to real community care has never been provided. Good support services demand reliability, as well as flexibility and co-operation across professional demarcation lines – often requiring a major shift in attitudes. A service provider writes: 'Flexibility is the key to designing good community based services. Traditionally services are designed around a building and staff – these can become ends in themselves . . . Community services are about turning the process upside down; starting with . . . what people need and . . . ways of meeting those needs' (Prins, 1990).

Some voluntary providers are developing this flexibility in their services (McEvoy, 1997). Some services now provide 'split' places (a time-shared arrangement) where two individuals with a disability spend half their time with their family and half in a community home. An ideology of informal family care as the ideal may avoid the grimness of institutional living and put a brake on requests for full-time substitute care, but it does not always enhance quality of life for either the disabled person or his/her carer. To request a full-time residential place can seem like a failure to cope; yet a minority of disabilities make care demands that are difficult to meet in a family context. 'Effective community care is dependent on the successful linking of both elements' (O'Connor, 1987) and this is not yet a reality.

Service provision: what is offered and who provides it?

Service provision in learning disability in Ireland is unique in that voluntary organisations are usually the providers, with the state's main role that of funder. Through the health boards, the state was also the provider of last resort and despite improvements, this sector has ended up with some of the least adequate services along with the neediest clients. Originally the main service providers in learning disability were religious orders and private charities, but since the 1960s provision has increasingly been undertaken by local parents' and friends' groups, which were set up to lobby for a service, but often ended up providing it. Involvement in provision can make lobbying more difficult.

The state's attitude towards the voluntary organisations has fluctuated. From the 1930s to the 1950s, service-provision by private charities seemed entirely natural and appropriate, with the state's only function to provide minor subvention; in the 1970s the state had embryonic plans for delivering services itself. Today, with the trend towards retrenching the scope of the state and with the influence of the privatisation of care services in the UK, the Irish state has a *de facto* policy of strengthening the role of the voluntary organisations in providing learning disability services, which it acknowledges as being to its benefit. The following quotation from the Department of Health's *Shaping a Healthier Future* (1994) paints the scenario at its ideal:

> The voluntary sector plays an integral role in the provision of health and personal social services . . . perhaps unparalleled in any other country. Traditionally, voluntary organisations have been to the forefront in identifying needs in the community and developing responses . . . Their independence enabled them to harness community support and to complement the statutory services in an innovative and flexible manner.

The community effort mobilised in starting a voluntary organisation and the social-action-type belief that it is better to light a candle than curse the darkness (or the government), are undoubtedly positive effects. So, too, is the relative independence of the voluntary organisations which gives them some leeway in using the media to raise the profile of people with disabilities, and to lobby for funding. Although some would argue that the agencies should have been more strident in this role, without their mediation learning disability was in constant danger of falling to the bottom of a health board's bag of priorities. Flexibility, a low level of bureaucracy and the ability to be innovative are other strengths of voluntary agencies. Nowadays, most funding comes from the Department of Health and Children (and to a lesser extent from the Department of Education and Science, and Department of Enterprise and Employment). In recent years most funds have been channelled through the health boards which enter into contracts with the larger voluntary organisations on services. The aim is to increase accountability, and to prevent jostling for funding between agencies. As levels of funding grow, partly because of the withdrawal of the religious orders, partly because care is of higher quality and continues for longer, Colgan (1997) quotes a tenfold increase over twenty years in the amounts spent on all types of disability – a greater degree of accountability is necessary. *Enhancing the Partnership* (Department of Health, 1997b), the report of the working group set up to iron out relationships between the learning disability providers and the state, broke new ground in setting out in a structured way relationships between the Department of Health and Children and the voluntary bodies. But the substantive issue – the issue of appropriate roles of the voluntary and statutory sectors in the provision of basic services has not yet been decided (Faughnan, 1997). Co-ordination, defined as 'systemic coherence running through the service system from its conception to its delivery' (Colgan, 1997: 11), is still at an initial stage in services for people with learning disabilities.

The existence of so many autonomous organisations (in *Enhancing Partnership* 14 are listed as directly funded by the Department of Health and Children, and there are others) gave rise in the past to fragmentation and rivalry, and seldom resulted in families or clients having a choice of service. Disability empires develop, rational planning is difficult and slow, and the voluntary organisations' ability to represent their clientele is dissipated. Whether a service is available in a locality may depend on whether the district had its own home-grown nineteenth-century philanthropist who donated land to a charity or religious order, or whether it had a group of committed middle-class parents thirty years ago. This leads to an uneven spread of facilities often favouring better-off and established communities. When funding was improved in 1998, it was notable that some voluntary organisations were much better able to seize this opportunity than were others; accordingly unevenness of provision may increase.

A second consideration is the issue of accountability and representation. Government expenditure is (eventually) audited; governments which misuse state funds can be voted out of office but similar provisions for voluntary organisations are patchy; some are responsible to their boards, some only to their religious superiors. Many voluntary organisations start off as an alliance of family and friends and they sometimes neglect to maintain representative structures; the trust or charity statutes under which they are established may make change cumbersome. A structure which suited a small, locally funded organisation needs to be remodelled when there is a budget of several million, most of it state-sourced.

Thirdly, although direct action to deal with a social problem can be an empowering option, it does allow the state to lay aside its underlying responsibility through apparently generous one-off contributions. A degree of buck-passing between state and voluntary body results in 'Catch 22' scenarios: parents pressurise agency to provide badly needed services; agency pleads lack of funds; parents approach government; government claims agency *has* sufficient funds; parents are unable to establish truth of either claim.

Finally, many voluntary bodies are set up in the heat of a pressing need and contain restrictions as to who may be 'helped'. Sometimes the very qualities which are a strength in setting up an organisation can be a disadvantage in the period of consolidation. Not every organisation has been able to change from the paternalistic connotation of 'help' to an emphasis on rights and ability, and there may be 'cherry-picking' of easier/more attractive clients who fit the social model. For example, providing new employment options for clients with a moderate learning disability and no behaviour problems may attract more funding, staff and laudatory comment than a support service for someone with multiple disabilities and behaviour problems.

Types of services

The major changes in services over the last 20 to 30 years have been the drop in residential placements, and the greater differentiation of day-services. The demand for out-of-home care for adults has meant that parents' and friends' groups originally set up to provide innovative day services are now attempting to develop small residential units. Most providers now have educational, training and employment branches.

The big changes in the education field are: (i) the move to integration, with more children with learning disabilities now attending national schools and some making their way through second-level schools; (ii) the increase in the number of training places which cater for the transitional stage between school and work, together with some training delivered by the mainstream service, FÁS; and (iii) the legal right to education whatever a child's disability. This was established by the O'Donoghue case (1996) in which a mother contested the state's refusal to give her a school place at the normal age, and when the High Court, and later the Supreme Court, found in favour of the child's right to an appropriate education, whatever his/her level of disability (Irish Court Reports, 1997, 2001).

The Sinnott case was for many a disappointment because it put an age limit rather than a need limit on educational provision, but it did challenge the strategy of the Department of Education and Science of saving by delay.[2] Provision of supports has increased considerably in recent years. The Education for Persons with Special Educational Needs Act 2004 covers assessment and review of need, individual educational plans, and it provides for a National Council for Special Education along with an appeals system. Importantly, it is based on children with disabilities having rights, though some groups

2   Kathryn Sinnott sought damages from the state on behalf of her son with autism because the education he had been offered was inadequate. She also sought to have educational provision made for him after age 18. She was awarded damages but, in the appeal by the Minister for Education and Science, the Supreme Court ruled that the state was not obliged to provide education for anyone over 18.

have contested its restrictive definitions – both of children and of educational disability.

Many parents are convinced that integrated schooling is the way forward, and the new Act is a major support for them. The necessary supports such as care assistants, resource teachers and equipment are appearing, with greater progress evident at primary than at secondary level. The establishment and planned expansion of NEPS (National Educational Psychological Services) and the National Council for Special Education (established under the Education for Persons with Special Educational Needs Act 2004) should make inroads into the waiting lists for assessments. It is important that a range of possible placements is available, including special schools and split schooling – half a week in a special school, the other half in the local school. Some services have set up ancillary supports for children in integrated education and this may be the way of the future. Although many children with severe and profound disabilities still go to day development centres, there are now provisions for teachers in these settings, improved pupil-teacher ratios and a National Council for Curriculum and Assessment (NCCA) committee has taken the first step on the matter of curriculum. In the future such children will probably receive their education in special schools. New thinking has also emerged in the education of children with autism, where the effectiveness of different methods has been strongly debated. The Department of Education and Science published a report in 2001. Large-scale research studies of outcomes in different types of schools will be needed to assess the outcomes of these changes.

Shortages in training places have caused crises for many young people with learning disabilities and their families. Planning to cater for the population bulge in the 20 to 34 age bracket has been slow, partly because this was the first cohort with learning disabilities to have a choice of opportunities in adulthood, partly because service providers sometimes held out for funding for an enhanced mix of services, rather than simply providing the old care-oriented model.

The fall in residential services has gone hand-in-hand with a much improved range of day services for adults. The prime mover was the EU programmes, Helios and Horizon, of the 1980s. Innovative programmes were also started to give part-time employment opportunities to people with severe learning disabilities who would earlier have been considered unsuitable. Sheltered workshops – the old model – became less popular with providers as the push for integrated open employment grew. While sheltered workshops have remained an important outlet for a large strand of people with disabilities, there have been considerable debates over their role, the boring nature of some of the contract work, and the rights, remuneration and needs of workers. Activation centres which provide sports and social programmes for adults who have part-time jobs in the community are another innovation. Although few people have gained employment steady and sufficiently well paid to allow them to come off social

welfare benefits, employment has added extra income and a degree of independence to the lives of many, as well as breaching attitudinal barriers among able-
bodied workers. The contradictions at the heart of the Disability Allowance –
that a recipient be permanently unable to work, apart from 'therapeutic'
employment – is an obstacle to greater participation in the labour market.
Separating the elements of the allowance into a pension (for those totally
unable to work) and a non-means-tested costs-of-disability allowance as suggested in *A Strategy for Equality* (Commission on the Status of People with
Disabilities, 1996) would be a useful way of addressing this problem.

Smaller-scale innovative services currently on offer include respite schemes,
which allow families of people with learning disabilities to have a break – holiday-
fostering schemes, friendship and leisure schemes (such as the volunteer-friend-
ship scheme initiated by Menni Enterprises (Kinsella, 1997)) – and within-service
advocacy training to give people the opportunity to speak for themselves, to
make choices. The Special Olympics – held in Ireland in 2003 – provided
another positive event which allowed people with learning disabilities to achieve
in an important media arena and involved the wider community in a very
positive way.

Consultation and representation

One of the most potent slogans of the disability movement has been: 'nothing
about us without us'. A major frustration for people with disabilities and their
families has been their lack of influence on the decisions affecting them. The
formation of the Commission on the Status of People with Disabilities, set up
under the Department of Equality and Law Reform in 1993, was a major
change: 60 per cent of its members were people with disabilities, their carers or
family members. The Commission also went to considerable pains to find out
people's opinions at listening meetings all over the country. Significantly, it
produced its findings in different formats – one version of its final report was
written for those with learning disabilities. Finding means of expression for
people with limited understanding of formal procedures is one of the challenges for this process.

The Council for People with Disabilities, which later became People with
Disabilities Ireland, now represents people with varying disabilities. Cross-
disability forums have become important both for lobbying and for understanding. The Commission's definition of disabled people included family
members (because they share in some of the disadvantage of disability), hence
family members as well as people with learning disability take part in these organisations. The National Disability Authority (NDA), established in 1998, also has
60 per cent representation of people with disabilities or their families on its board.

Bodies whose decisions materially affect the lives of people with disabilities need to build in more consultation. *Enhancing the Partnership* (Department of Health, 1997b) recommended developing 'mechanisms for consulting persons with mental handicap and their families' but insufficient representation on health board planning committees continued. Equality proofing – looking at all policies for their impact on people with disabilities – requires representation. As McConkey and Conliffe (1989: 4) put it 'Effective planning involves more than counting heads or beds. People's needs, wishes and aspirations need to be taken into account.' Voluntary groups also need to ensure that channels between management and users and their families are kept open. The philosophical orientation of the Disability Bill 2001 (which was duty rather than rights-based) and the response which it met from disabled people's groups are evidence that such consultation must be more than skin-deep. The campaign, led by a coalition of different disability groups, also marked the major maturing of these organisations since *A Strategy for Equality*. With the Freedom of Information Act, the culture of hierarchy and unexplained decisions in Irish official life has begun to change but a culture of true and equal partnership has not yet taken its place.

Future directions in policy for people with learning disabilities

The recommendations of *A Strategy for Equality* have been accepted in principle; the Employment Equality Act and the Equal Status Act are now law; a second Disability Bill has been published and an Education for Persons with Special Educational Needs Act has been passed; the Equality Authority, the National Disability Authority and Comhairle (the information, advice and advocacy agency) have been set up and resourced. There was a major increase in funding for disability services between 1998 and 2001 (though it was not proportionate to Ireland's astonishing economic growth); structures in voluntary agencies are improving. A child with the most severe disability now has a right to an education; in many supermarkets and offices, young people with a learning disability find part-time work. These are all advances.

The immediate challenge undoubtedly lies in the development and funding of high quality residential places in the community for the bulge generation of those in the 20 to 30 age group, most of whom will eventually lose their parents and their original homes. An article in *Rett News* (a UK journal) described a successful care plan which one family had set up for their severely disabled adult daughter. Adjacent to the family's home, a small bungalow was built, which their daughter purchased under a shared ownership scheme. Six care assistants were employed to care for the woman in 'a supported homely environment;' the costs were met by the local authority and the British Social Fund, and were no greater than her former residential care package (Ormian and Ormian, 1998). A similar Irish scheme catering for people with much greater independence required a considerable subvention from families (Clarke, 1990). Service brokerage, direct payments and a range of choices have not yet come to Ireland, yet some of the community homes set up by voluntary organisations now provide a fulfilling life for adults with learning disabilities.

Maintaining quality in services is another key area and some service providers are addressing it. The National Disability Authority is also piloting quality standards in residential care institutions and a system of inspection may be introduced under the advocacy and review procedures in the new disability legislation. An independent complaints system is essential, as individuals and families can have difficulties making a case to a service provider on whom they are dependent. Although agencies and staff generally have shown a high standard of service and dedication, experience in child care and in some psychiatric hospitals has demonstrated the necessity of independent monitoring. Advocacy and self-advocacy services are also essential: this is one of the areas addressed in the Disability Bill and Comhairle Amendment Bill 2004.

Guardianship legislation for those with limited capacity to take decisions for themselves is also overdue, as a publication by NAMHI (2003) suggests. The present legal position on some sensitive medical and financial issues affecting people with learning disabilities (consent to treatment, right to contraception, requirement of disclosure to parents, sterilisation) is unclear.

Government departments need to find ways to encourage innovative programmes and research, for it would be arrogant to suppose that the high-water-mark in wisdom about learning disability has been reached. In particular, the range of support services must increase. In the area of education for children with severe and profound disabilities, specialised training for teachers is particularly urgent.

There are four signs I shall be looking for to see if Ireland is serious about treating people with learning disability as equal citizens. Will the mental handicap Wards in St Ita's, Portrane finally close? Will it be normal to find a couple of people with learning disabilities in most workplaces? Will families be given a range of placements for an adult with learning disabilities at a time of their choosing? And will there be a monitoring and complaints system for disability services?

Editor's Addenda

Expenditure Estimates 2004
In November 2004, the Minister for Finance, Brian Cowen, in publishing the Expenditure Estimates, indicated that some €2.8 billion overall would be provided in 2005, especially for people with disabilities – an increase of 11 per cent on the 2004 figure. In his Budget speech, on 1 December 2004, he announced that the €2.8 billion would fund: health sector services specifically for people with an intellectual disability or autism, physical or sensory disabilities, and mental illness; first-, second- and third-level special needs education; specialised training and employment support services provided by FÁS; the cost of certain tax reliefs to assist mobility; and the adaptation of accommodation specifically for persons with disabilities.

Further, the minister estimated that by the end of 2009, as a result of increased funding, over 4,500 extra residential, respite and day places would be provided for persons with an intellectual, physical or sensory disability or autism; about 600 persons with intellectual disability or autism would be transferred out of psychiatric hospitals and other inappropriate places; about 1.2 million extra hours of home support and personal assistance would be provided for persons with physical or sensory disabilities; and 400 new places would be provided in community-based mental health facilities. Groups representing people with disabilities broadly welcomed the planned funding increases. The extent to which these measures, when implemented, will help resolve the many issues raised in chapters 11 and 12 remains to be seen.

Disability Act 2005
In September 2004, a long-awaited Disability Bill was published by the government. In the bill, disability was defined as an impairment resulting in a substantial restriction in the capacity of a person to carry on a profession, business or occupation, or to participate in social or cultural life. A person so defined would have his or her educational and health needs appraised by an assessment officer who would have an independent statutory function. A statement of the services considered appropriate for the person would also be provided along with a timescale for their delivery. Crucially, it was indicated that the service statement would take into account the availability of financial resources. The procedure for accessing services did not include resort to the courts. Instead, the bill set out a rather complex complaints and appeals system, with the right to the assistance of an advocate supplied by Comhairle. The bill also obliged public bodies to make their public buildings accessible to all, and gave a statutory basis to the requirement that they implement a target of three per cent for employing people with disabilities. Despite its rejection as inadequate by organisations representing people with disabilities, the bill was passed into law in May 2005.

Chapter 12

People with physical disability: health policy and practice

Anne Colgan

People with physical disabilities, and those who are active in promoting ideals of equality and full participation for and with them, may well question why a publication on health policy contains a chapter concerned with health policy issues for people with physical disabilities. Why should they, as a sector of the community, warrant specific consideration?

The justification arises firstly from the fact that people with disabilities are a significant group of users of the health services, as those services are currently constituted. For most adults and children with physical disabilities, the disability is almost invariably connected to a point in time or to a period of time, or even recurring events, when disability manifests itself as illness, requiring diagnosis, treatment and perhaps ongoing medical care and support. Surgical intervention, pain management, prescription of medication, ongoing consultation and access to medical rehabilitation tend to feature in the lives of people with physical disabilities. A study carried out by the National Rehabilitation Board (NRB) showed that, in the twelve-month period prior to the study, just under two thirds of disabled people interviewed had visited their doctor. More than one third had spent time in hospital (NRB, 1993). Given this level of involvement with the health (treatment) services, there is a case for exploring the extent to which health policy responds to the specific health care needs of people with disabilities.

A further dimension of health policy in its relationship with people with physical disabilities stems from the wider role of health services as providers of personal social services. This kind of provision has been a feature of Irish health services from a very early point in their development, and people with physical disabilities have been significant users of these services. For example, provision for income maintenance for people with a disability was first introduced in the 1954 Health Act. The administration of Disabled Persons Maintenance Allowance, which was introduced at that point was transferred to the Department of Social Welfare and the Family only in 1997. Training and employment provisions for people with disabilities have also been the responsibility of the Department of Health, with the health boards having the executive responsibility for training and employment services since their inception through the 1970 Health Act. A very significant range of personal support services such as personal assistance, respite care services, day activity services, technical aids and appliances, continue to be part of the remit of the health services. Policy in respect of this form of provision impacts very strongly on the lives of people with physical disabilities.

A second, broader, justification for examining health service policy in relation to people with physical disabilities, linked to the issues of provision which have just been described, arises from the wider need to explore the interaction between health policy and the sociology of disability. To what extent and in what ways has health policy, and the infrastructures through which that policy is linked to practice, shaped the experience of people with disabilities? What public perception of disability has health service policy helped to create? From a systemic perspective, how has health policy and its delivery structure interacted with other dimensions of public policy to create a social construct of disability? The issues and considerations that arise are not unique to people with physical disabilities. However, it is reasonable to contend that it is in the lives of people with physical disabilities that these issues are made very explicitly real in the widest possible range of areas of daily living, and that people with physical disabilities have led the challenge for change to new models and constructs of disability.

The conceptual framework

Consideration of health policy in its relationship to people with physical disability opens up a tangled web of historical, cultural, political, social and administrative facets of the issue, thus underlining the complex sociological framework within which the corpus of policy rests. In-depth consideration of all of these interplays over time and in their wider international context would not be feasible here. However, as a context for exploring and making observa - tions on Irish health policy, they must at least be acknowledged. Oliver (1990) engages in a wide-ranging analysis of these many facets of the understanding of disability in the task he undertook – that of beginning to apply sociological perspectives to the issue of disability. Oliver examines, in historical terms, the manner in which major economic and social movements such as the rise of capitalism and the development of the welfare state shaped the experience of people with disabilities; he explores cultural phenomena of stigma, and medical and psychological models of 'adjustment'. He looks at the sub-groups within the wider grouping of people with disabilities, such as women and black people. He explains his aims:

It is not the intention to use the category of disability to resolve disputes within sociology itself, whether they be about economic determinism, relative autonomy, ideology or whatever else. Rather the intention is more limited; to show that disability as a category can only be understood within a framework, which suggests that it is culturally produced and socially structured (Oliver, 1990: 22).

One specific and very central focus of the analysis of the understandings of disability, and what is perceived as the consequential structuring of policy and practice, is the tension between the medical and social models of disability. This proposed tension has very particular meaning and significance for people with physical disabilities, since it is in their experience and in their lives that the conflation of illness, requiring diagnosis and treatment, and disability, requiring social responses, has been most compelling.

As part of its work for the Commission on the Status of People with Disabilities, the Commission's Working Group on Health (1996) considered the importance of perceptions of the operation of the medical/social model in the Irish context. The tendency for an unhelpful polarisation of the issues was noted by the Working Group:

> Interwoven with this debate about differing philosophies of care are agendas relating to differing professional systems models competing for dominance in the health care system. Furthermore, alongside the traditional clinical professionals is a new grouping which is gaining an increasingly powerful role in this system – that of administrative professionals who are faced with the organisation and measurement of resource inputs and outputs to satisfy both government and public. Therefore the first step in this analysis is to appreciate the complexity of the system and to recognise that, because of these various agendas, there is a tendency . . . to polarise issues and models as various professions identify with different models of care (Working Group on Health, 1996: 22).

The Working Group identified the medical model of care as one deriving more broadly from a clinical or pathological model, involving diagnosis and treatment. It is seen as a 'deficit' model, where the 'deficit' is intrinsic to the person, and which may be amenable to treatment and cure. The model is also seen as descriptive in the context of the interaction between people with disabilities and a wide range of professionals – therapists, psychologists, teachers – and not only doctors. In fact, it could be argued that the medical model legitimately applies to the doctor–patient relationship, which is quite valid at certain points in the life of a person with a physical disability, as in the case of every person. The difficulty arises when the doctor–patient model of relationship is transferred beyond the period of illness to other facets of living, and when other professionals adopt the model, with its implications for a strong imbalance of power in the relationship. The social model, as described by the Working Group, acknowledges the handicapping effects of a society geared to 'ablebodiedness' as the norm:

> This model theoretically shifts the focus from the disability to the person, views disability as a social creation and rejects the notion that a person can be defined by a condition which affects them (Working Group on Health, 1996: 26).

It was clear from the submissions received by the Commission that many Irish people with disabilities reject a medical model, and the linked concept of rehabilitation which has been the bedrock of policy in respect of people with disabilities in Ireland. The concept of 'rehabilitation' found its expression in the Health Acts, and was institutionalised in the names and assigned roles of key organisations in the disability field, such as the National Rehabilitation Board (set up in 1963) and the National Medical Rehabilitation Centre, set up to provide treatment and care for people who have suffered spinal injuries. Of course, it must be said that concepts such as rehabilitation were products of their time; they reflected best current thinking in their time.

The Working Group acknowledged that the term and concept of the medical model is used often in an ill-defined way, which may unfairly categorise the spectrum of medical thinking and unfairly generalise about the practice of individual doctors. It has become in some senses a cypher for dissatisfactions with disempowering professional practices in general and with policies, including health policy, which retain an emphasis on care, and resist a systemic approach, involving the building of an inclusive, holistic response to disability. In the following sections, it is proposed to look at some dimensions of Irish health policy, and related structures and practices against the background of the debate on conceptual frameworks and models of provision.

The data on physical disability

It is usual when exploring any area of public policy in respect of a specific group of people to attempt to define as precisely as possible the number of people to whom that policy area applies. Our capacity to understand the issues, or to propose solutions, seems to depend in some measure on having a 'picture' of the numbers of people involved and their 'characteristics'. This very strong need to count, categorise and classify is in itself a critical sociological phenomenon in respect of people with physical disabilities, integrally linked to the ideological issues raised in the previous section.

The need to count, classify and categorise may well be a powerful intuitive need into which we have been socialised, as a way of making sense of particular social experiences. However, the more specific practical justification is an administrative one, related to the need to measure and plan for resource allocation. This, in turn, it has been argued, links systemically with a welfare-based model of support for people with disabilities, in which the definition of disability is intrinsically linked with categories of eligibility for services provided by or through the state. Where resources are not unlimited (as is generally the case), approaches to defining entitlement are likely to be influenced by the question of how many people may be eligible for a particular service; eligibility, in turn, tends to create the framework for 'counting' the numbers of people with disability – thus creating an administrative and self-perpetuating circularity.

Oliver (1990) places this issue in an international historical context. He draws on the work of Stone (1984), who has observed that in the late twentieth century, standards of eligibility for services had become extremely detailed, in turn resulting in more inflexible categories of disability and rigid resource led concepts of disability which were internalised by disabled people themselves:

> Once certain groups are accepted into the category, they cannot be ejected from it; people become socialised into their role as 'disabled', and disability categoris-ation is legitimised by the medical and welfare bureaucracies (Oliver, 1990: 42).

All of these phenomena can be observed at work in the Irish context. As part of its work, the Commission on the Status of People with Disabilities examined in depth the question of statistical data relating to the numbers of people with disabilities in Ireland. The Commission outlined clearly the reasons why the task of 'counting' people with disabilities (and, in particular, people with physical disabilities) is fraught with difficulty. The first difficulty is that which has already been identified as a serious philosophical issue in the discussion on conceptual frameworks: the approach to the definition of disability, and whether it is based on a medical or social definition. The Commission lists other difficulties: the relative nature of the concept of disability; the difficulty in distinguishing between illness and disability; prevailing concepts of 'normality'; the overlap between people with disabilities and elderly people (Commission on the Status of People with Disabilities, 1996).

In spite of these difficulties, the Commission sought to secure the best possible estimates of the number of people with disabilities in Ireland, based on work done on their behalf by the Economic and Social Research Institute. This work estimates the overall number of people with disabilities at 360,000, or 10 per cent of the population. The Commission acknowledges that these are conservative estimates. People with physical disabilities are estimated to account for 50 to 80 per cent of the total numbers, with those with locomotor impair-ments predominating in the group. In the course of their work, the Review Group on Health and Personal Social Services for People with Physical and

Sensory Disabilities (Review Group, 1996) struggled with this issue, specifically as it related to people with physical and sensory disabilities. Like the Commission, and indeed virtually every other government report on aspects of disability policy, the Review Group noted the lack of data on the numbers and service needs of people with physical and sensory disabilities. The Report went on to develop its own estimates of the prevalence of disability, based largely on extrapolations from the 1988 survey carried out by the British Office of Population Censuses and Surveys (OPCS). Using these extrapolations, the Report estimated a total number of people with physical and sensory disability at 109,300 – a significantly lower figure than that produced by the Commission.

In framing its recommendations for a national database, the Review Group acknowledged that studies of prevalence gave no indication of actual health service needs. They recommended the establishment of a database which would meet the need for incidence and prevalence figures, but which would also contain information on service needs, of a sufficiently reliable quality to allow for long-term planning of service provision. This task was given to a National Physical and Sensory Disability Database Committee, set up in 1998. Work on the development of the database has been ongoing for several years, operating at health board level.

The intractability of the data issue, especially in the case of people with physical disabilities, is directly related to the question of how needs are determined. The task of developing a database in respect of people with physical disabilities has been bedevilling health service administrators for almost twenty years. The health boards, in partnership with the National Rehabilitation Board, were initially given this task in 1981. Reports on the outcome indicate a range of barriers, including the non-availability of staffing at health board level. However, the more fundamental difficulty is the fact that, in the case of people with physical disability, service need cannot be inferred from the diagnostic label that the person happens to wear. Individual capacities, motivations, family supports, access to education, will all shape the way in which the individual interacts with the functional impairment resulting from the disability. The process of determining need, then, is a complex process which must take account not only of all these factors, but also of the specific local environment in which the person operates. In this process of needs identification, the tensions between medical and social model become very real indeed.

Policy making and service delivery

Oliver (1990) explores the extent to which public policy can create an ideological construction of disability, arguing that these policies themselves are usually based on implicit ideologies which are rarely the subject of rigorous analysis. These policies and underpinning ideologies find expression in the institutional arrangements for policy making, for funding and for service delivery. The two most significant facets of the institutional arrangements, from the perspective of people with physical disabilities are, firstly, the distribution of policy responsibility among government departments, and secondly, the distribution of responsibility and resources for service delivery between the voluntary sector organisations and the state – a facet of organisational arrangements which has hugely significant implications in the Irish context.

Distribution of departmental responsibilities

From the foundation of the state, responsibility for policy and services for people with disabilities had been located within the Department of Health. The introduction of the Disabled Person's Maintenance Allowance in 1953 was undoubtedly an important step in enabling people with disabilities to have some measure of financial security and independence. However, the locating of responsibility for this and a number of other income maintenance provisions for people with disabilities within the ambit of the health services laid the groundwork for a heavily medicalised approach to income maintenance for people with disabilities. This arrangement may have contributed to a climate of low expectations among people with disabilities that they could hope to gain employment or attempt training for employment. The health service based arrangements for income maintenance were structurally linked to the health service based system for offering employment and training opportunities to people with disabilities. These systems and structures have involved a network of institutional arrangements involving the health boards, the Department of Health, the National Rehabilitation Board (set up under the Health, Corporate Bodies Act 1963) and a network of voluntary service providers.

The impact of this strongly health-focused and separate provision for basic services for people with disabilities were underlined and supplemented by the fact that other major service providing government departments and their agencies, responsible for areas such as transport, physical access, employment, training, housing, did not have a legal remit or a formalised policy responsibility for meeting the access, housing or employment needs of people with disabilities. This has had particular significance for people with physical disabilities, for whom access, transport, accessible housing provision and access to mainstream training services are critical to inclusion in their local community.

One of the outcomes of this compartmentalisation of service delivery into the health field over the past fifty years was its impact on funding strategies. Government departments, having no formalised responsibility to ensure access to these mainstream services for people with disabilities, did not have to budget for such provision; there was no requirement, over the years, to make fiscal arrangements for accessible transport, for accessible public offices for government departments, for widely accessible local authority housing. Thus the funding for any developments in these areas had to be borne by the health services in its networks of special provisions rather than being seen and operated as an integral social cost for all government departments. The exception to this pattern has been the provision of education services for children with disabilities, which has been within the remit of the Department of Education, albeit mainly provided through special schools, and with significant inputs from the health services for residential provision and the provision of support services such as psychological and clinical services.

This is not to suggest that the mainstream providers of public services have not engaged at all with the provision of services for people with physical disabilities. For example, a wide range of initiatives to promote access to public buildings has been taken by the Department of the Environment over the years, such as the introduction of building regulations requiring all new buildings to adhere to specifications making them accessible to people with physical and other disabilities (Department of the Environment, 1991). However, such initiatives have mainly been the outcome of the promotional work of the National Rehabilitation Board since it was set up in 1963. The value and worth of these initiatives did not take away from the reality of the central structural feature of policy and service delivery structures for core public services until very recently – their concentration within the health services in the case of people with physical and other disabilities – and the importance of that for the way people with disabilities have been perceived, and served.

State–voluntary sector relationship

The strong involvement of voluntary organisations in the delivery of health services has been one of the most marked features of health service provision in Ireland:

> The voluntary sector plays an integral role in the provision of health and personal social services in Ireland which is probably unparalleled in any other country. Traditionally, voluntary organisations have been to the forefront in identifying needs in the community and in developing responses to them (Department of Health, 1994a).

The Department of Health's 1994 strategy document, *Shaping A Healthier Future*, acknowledged the significance of the role of the voluntary sector, and the ways in which its independence had enabled it to engage in innovation and in flexible responses to emerging needs. What has been the impact for people with physical disabilities of the strong voluntary sector role in service provision in relation to health and personal social services? Pauline Faughnan pointed to the absence of a clear framework for the state–voluntary sector relationship:

> Despite the importance of the activities of the voluntary sector and the role it has traditionally played in Irish society, there is no policy at national level within which its contribution may be located. There is no clear statement of principles which underlie the relationship between the voluntary and statutory sectors in general. (Faughnan, 1997: 238)

Faughnan went on to outline the manner in which the absence of such a framework has resulted in denying to the voluntary sector an appropriate role in policy-making:

> For a long time the voluntary and community sectors, while seeking partnership with Government departments and state agencies, have not been included in policy-making. Existing consultation processes were recently described by the National Economic and Social Forum as limited, reactive and unsatisfactory (Faughnan, 1997: 239).

There is a question as to whether this analysis applies fully to the voluntary sector providing services to people with disabilities. It can be argued that in the learning disability field in particular, the voluntary agencies have had a very strong role in shaping provision, and that policy has, in effect, equalled provision; learning disability services have, since the foundation of the state, been provided mainly by the major mental handicap organisations, rather than by the state, and the pattern of development has been one in which services have been initiated by the voluntary sector, with the state providing the funding. The 'battle' for that funding to meet the identified need has tended to be the main focus of the agencies and departmental policy has tended to be developed through the medium of working parties and commissions set up from time to time to examine service provision. These working parties have been exceedingly influential in shaping policy and services. The voluntary sector has been strongly represented on these working parties. Early examples of such influential short-term bodies have been the 1965 Commission of Enquiry on Mental Handicap, which exerted an enduring influence on all aspects of service structure within mental handicap services, and the 1974 Report on the Training and Employment of the Handicapped.

It is perhaps through the arrangements for funding of service delivery that the greatest impact of the various relationships between the statutory health agencies and the voluntary sector can be seen. Faughnan remarked that 'the funding systems within which voluntary organisations operated in the health arena were, with a few notable exceptions, fragmented, insecure and short term' (Faughnan, 1997: 242). This applied most particularly, however, to the smaller organisations operating on the basis of discretionary grant aid from the health boards, and these were mainly organisations working with and for people with physical disability. Organisations in the learning disability fields have for the most part been directly funded on a budgetary basis by the Department of Health, thus generating greater security of funding, and more direct and ready influence on funding allocation. The grant-aided bodies, on the other hand, have experienced funding arrangements which were 'uncertain, insecure and sometimes inappropriate . . . and militating against good management because of delays in payment and their year to year basis' (Faughnan, 1997: 242).

Organisations for and of people with physical disability have tended to be smaller, more fragmented and more vulnerable in relation to funding and influence, compared with the strongly organised service providers in the learning disability sector. There is a commonly held perception that learning disability services have tended to fare much better in funding arrangements than the physical disability sector. And it is noteworthy, for example, that it has been the learning disability sector, through their umbrella organisation for service providers, which has led the way in forging a new form of agreement concerning the structuring of contractual arrangements for service provision between their sector and the Department of Health.

The reasons for the apparent fragmentation of voluntary organisations in the physical disability field are complex. The range of organisations reflects the wide range of kinds of disability; each of these represents a very different kind of life experience on the part of those with that disability. Stroke survivors, people with epilepsy, families of young people with muscular dystrophy – there may be unifying experiences, but there are also dimensions of living with the disability that are particular. People want and are entitled to share their particular experience. The small disability organisations make that possible: they can bring together peer groups for critical peer support, and they can highlight the special concerns of people arising from their particular experience of their disability. This diversity has undoubtedly been needed and wanted by people with physical disability themselves. The 'downside' of this diversity is that it is difficult for these small organisations to put in place a significant organisational infrastructure and to command the resources to do so, particularly outside major urban areas. There is huge reliance on volunteers – a factor which is part of their strength but also one which makes them vulnerable. There is a real fear that, in the organisational and funding arrangements, the value and worth of these small groups will be overlooked, that they will be seen as 'inefficient'. Organisational arrangements for regional co-ordinating committees with a remit in partnering the health boards in planning and co-ordination of services may have tended to give primacy to the large, strong voluntary sector. Smaller organisations delivering a range of flexible personal supports may be more vulnerable as a result, continuing to depend on discretionary grant aid. Thus it presents a real challenge for the umbrella organisation, of which most of these groups are members, the Disability Federation of Ireland, to ensure, with them, that their significant place in the spectrum of support for people with physical disabilities is maintained and strengthened.

Thrust of future policy and provision

While the focus of policy in the past has been on service provision and, in particular, the provision of caring services, the pressure now is for the new focus of policy to be towards the building of equality, full participation, independence and inclusion. In the wider social context, the movement is towards a civil rights focus on disability issues; there is an emphasis on legislative provision for equality and full participation. This development is deeply rooted in international developments, and supported by the work of respected international bodies – in particular the United Nations and the European Union. In legislative terms, the lead has been given by the Americans with the Disabilities Act, which has consolidated and developed a strong anti-discrimination focus in American legislation and policy. This legislation is being used as a model for anti-discrimination in several countries. Many of its key elements and definitions were included in legislative proposals adopted by the Commission on the Status of People with Disabilities.

One of the most significant international measures influencing thinking in Ireland and elsewhere has been the preparation and dissemination of the UN Standard Rules for the Equalisation of Opportunities for Persons with Disabilities, adopted by the UN in 1993. Although these Rules are not legally binding on UN member states, they are of strong moral and practical significance:

> these Rules provide a legal standard for programmes, policies and laws which address the issue of full participation and equality for people with disabilities. They are of immense significance in that they provide specific targets for participation across the spectrum of aspects of daily living, thus offering ready-made performance indicators for any government seriously committed to the task of securing inclusion and participation. (Colgan, 1997: 123)

Already, in the Irish context, the Rules are being actively drawn into the policy-making process. They constitute the framework for the agreement which has been drawn up between the Department of Health and Children and the Federation of Voluntary Bodies Providing Services for People with Mental Handicap. This agreement sets out the terms of service contracts between the state and voluntary service providers in the learning disabilities field. Its terms are likely to become the norm for service contracts in the physical disabilities services.

The Standard Rules have also influenced European Union thinking, and they were reflected in an important new draft resolution from the Council of Ministers, published in December 1996. The language of that directive signals very strongly the shift in emphasis from a dependency model of service to an independence model with a much wider social focus stretching way beyond the health field. The European Commission states that the stereotyping of people with disabilities, the prejudicial attitudes which they experience, and the 'self-perpetuating cycle of exclusion' have all been compounded by the absence of people with disabilities from mainstream services (European Commission, 1996: 7). So the emphasis in the debate about good ways of meeting special concerns is shifting to embody wider issues about social participation and inclusion. The emphasis now is on a human and civil rights approach.

People with physical disabilities have been to the forefront in bringing forward the new thinking. Oliver (1990) traces the history of the disability movement as a new social movement, with its reflection in similar movements of black people and women, and the related shift towards an anti-discrimination focus. The Independent Living Movement in the United States began as early as the 1960s, with the development of Independent Living centres run by people with disabilities themselves. Internationally, the strong symbol of change, in that and following decades, has been the wish and will of people with disabilities (with people with physical disabilities in the forefront) to run their own organisations, rather than to be served by organisations *for* people with disabilities; that disabled people should take control of their own lives and make their own decisions as to how their needs can best be met. This author was present in Toronto at the 1980 Congress of Rehabilitation International, the international federation of organisations working in the field of disability, when that organisation rejected a proposal from disabled people present to translate itself into an organisation *of* people with disability. The decision led to the formation of an embryonic new organisation, Disabled People International, which has now become a significant player in the international disability movement. The 'revolution' in Toronto was actively promoted and prompted by an Irishman, the late Liam Maguire, himself a wheelchair user following a car accident.

As a committed trade unionist, Liam Maguire managed to put disability issues firmly on the agenda of the Irish Congress of Trade Unions. In doing so, he set an important precedent that has influenced and shaped developments right up to the present day. As national agreements have become the norm, and the successive agreements of government and the social partners have become a very significant determinant of social policy in a whole range of areas, Liam Maguire's legacy has been that the Irish Congress of Trade Unions has continued to be a major advocate for change, inclusion and investment in services for people with disabilities. The disability issue is always on the national agenda, even if many activists would be dissatisfied with the pace of progress. Perhaps one may identify here a significant prerequisite of securing change – that people with disabilities ally themselves with a powerful mainstream group with political influence who will advocate alongside them.

In Ireland, as in other countries, new movements of people with disabilities have emerged over two decades. The first of these, the Forum of People with Disabilities, was particularly influential in securing from the then Taoiseach, Albert Reynolds, a commitment for the setting up of the Commission on the Status of People with Disabilities, and a commitment for the establishment of a permanent Council of People with Disabilities. The Commission's report, published in 1997, has been accepted as the basis for the development of national disability policy, and the Council, People with Disabilities Ireland (PwDI), is now in place.

Challenges in the development of participation and inclusion

Structures and frameworks are being built which are more in tune with these policy developments. As these begin to be put in place, what are the major barriers to participation and inclusion at the present time? As part of its work, the Commission on the Status of People with Disabilities set out to answer this. While many reports and review bodies had identified future directions, people with disabilities themselves had never been asked for their perspective in a systematic way. It was part of the ethos of the Commission that it should do so, rather than presume to know. 'Listening meetings' were held throughout the country. People with disabilities were actively encouraged to write, send tapes or call the Commission on its freephone telephone lines. Special arrangements were made to hear from groups who might be marginalised in large public meetings – young people with disabilities, people with mental health difficulties, Travellers with disabilities, women with disabilities, gay and lesbian people with disabilities. The outcome was a comprehensive and unique critique of current policies. While a full account of the outcome cannot be included here, the thrust and direction of the findings are significant in terms of health policy and its relationship to wider social policy.

A qualitative analysis was carried out of the 504 written submissions to the Commission, the majority of which came from people with physical disabilities. This analysis showed that people were expressing their concerns, not so much in terms of gaps in services, but in terms of the sense of frustration, marginalisation and stress they were experiencing as a result of the many deficits in opportunities for a reasonable quality of life:

One of the most striking features of the submissions as a whole was the sense of absolute frustration which emerged from them. The frustration did not centre, as some might expect, on personal experiences of physical pain, discomfort or impaired function. On the contrary, the frustration which was articulated revolved around people's sense that they were being put in a position of having to deal with a myriad of oppressive social barriers in addition to their disabling conditions (Tubridy, 1995: 6).

Access to the built environment and accessible transport topped the league table of issues raised in written submissions, followed by education and income support (Cousins, 1995). This is hardly surprising since, for people with physical disability in particular, these four features of daily living, in this order, shape in the most direct and tangible possible way their opportunities for participation and inclusion. The fragmentation of service delivery and the lack of a single point of contact and a single process for assessment of entitlement and for information provision were priority issues raised by people with disabilities. It is noteworthy that health services, in the narrow sense of medical services, was low on the list of issues, with the focus there on medical cards, entitlements for access to medical and surgical appliances, access to hospitals and surgeries and the need for specialised services for specific groups, such as those who have experienced brain injury.

One of the most powerful messages coming across from the listening meetings held by the Commission, as well as from written submissions, was the central importance of access to information – information about rights and entitlements, information about services, options and choices, information about disability. This fact (and the response which is taken to it) highlights in a very particular way the need for a shift from a model of policy and service delivery where providers are central, to one where people with disabilities themselves have a measure of control over their lives. Choice presupposes information. Information about entitlements and rights presumes that there are entitlements and rights. At an even more basic level, information provision, in formats accessible to the public, is resource intensive. Power and influence can be managed by those who hold, and can withhold, information. Its provision, or rather its absence, as far as public services in general are concerned, has been strongly criticised by the National Economic and Social Forum (NESF, 1995).

Information provision is not value-free. Where the control of information rests with service providers, they tend to tell people what they, the professionals, assume people with disabilities need to know. Not only the policy in respect of information provision, but also the precise manner of delivering on the policy will be critical to whether the policy proves to be a genuinely empowering one:

Disability information is based on a disabled experience. For example, the information about how people with personal assistance needs can function as full citizens can be summed up in the words 'independent living'. This concept did not exist until disabled people invented it. We could not have asked non-disabled people for this information – they could not create it because they do not have a disabled consciousness. If the information we are given does not start from a disabled viewpoint it is not the information we need. (Hasler, 1993:11)

The challenge of developing person-centred information systems now rests primarily with Comhairle, the statutory authority with overall responsibility for public information, as well as with individual agencies, health boards and government departments, who must look critically at their own information delivery practices in the light of the new focus on empowerment.

The role of needs assessment

One of the critical processes which will determine whether there is genuine empowerment of people with physical disabilities and others will be the process within the health system (and other systems) for the identification of need. This process is value laden. It can be structured in a way that places a premium on professional assessment, professional language, professional perspectives on personal priorities, or it can balance those essential inputs with the views, wishes and perspectives of those who own the needs – the people with disabilities, their families and carers. This is a key process, at the heart of planning and implementation of policy. A social model of disability would require professionals to share power with disabled people in the assessment of need. New processes of measuring need would acknowledge that disabled people are experts in their own lives and their own needs. It is only when these tools of the system are refashioned that policy, built on the accumulated information about individual needs, can be truly seen to be responsive and reflective of those needs.

The legislative framework for future directions

More than anything else, the legislative framework is seen as creating a powerful context that shapes and directs policy, determines the focus of service delivery structures, and embodies an expression of the way in which people with disabilities are viewed both as citizens and as service users. Since the publication of the Report of the Commission on the Status of People with Disabilities in 1996, some foundational pieces of legislation have been passed which have had profound significance for people with disabilities. The Equal

Status Act 1996 and the Education Act 1998, for example, are notable for the fact that they address the disability issues as part of mainstream legislative provision. While the Education of Persons with Special Needs Act 2004 makes specific legislative provision for the education of people with special needs, the focus of the Act is on ensuring the students with special needs can participate in mainstream educational services. Thus we are seeing a seismic shift in the way in which the framework of legislative provision for people with disabilities has moved from the specialist to mainstream, inclusive legislation, and has become the province and responsibility of each government department.

One of the core recommendations of the Commission on the Status of People with Disabilities was that disability legislation should be enacted which would set out the rights of people with disabilities and means of redress for those whose rights are denied. A Disabilities Bill, outlining a statutory framework for the assessment of need and provision of services, was published in 2001, following lengthy consultation with people with disabilities and advocacy organisations. This Bill was strongly opposed by virtually all of the advocacy organisations, and was subsequently withdrawn by government. The Bill was perceived to have several fundamental weaknesses. The lack of a rights-based approach to services and the dependence of service provision on the availability of resources rather than an entitlement based on assessed need were features most strongly opposed by the disability sector. The Bill also sought to limit access to the courts in pursuit of a right to services, another element that led to its rejection.

Following the withdrawal of that Bill, an unprecedented consultation process took place between civil society stakeholders and government. This consultative process culminated in the publication of the Disability Bill 2004. This Bill is complex and multi-faceted. It provides for a broad national disability strategy, of which the arrangements for service provision are but one part. It requires key government departments to produce sectoral plans for people with disability; it places a legal obligation on public bodies to employ people with disabilities; access to public buildings and access to information – two core aspects of ensuring participation in all aspects of social living – are covered in the Bill. On the needs/service delivery side, the Bill provides a framework for independent needs assessment, and a service statement, together with arrangements for a complex set of complaints and appeals procedures; a personal advocacy service, and a mediation service may be provided to assist a person who wishes to challenge the outcome of the needs assessment, or the implementation of the service statement. The legislation thus adopts a two-pronged approach, providing for mainstream responsibility to include people with disabilities, while also acknowledging that disabled people have many additional support needs that must be met in order for them to participate on equal terms. In its provisions, the Bill would appear to address many of the

critical dimensions of provision for inclusion identified by people with disabilities and described so clearly in their feedback to the Commission on the Status
of People with Disabilities. Notwithstanding this, and the extensive consultation
which preceded it, the Bill has met with mixed reaction, ranging from warm
welcome to outright rejection as fundamentally flawed. Reservations about the
Bill focus on the continued linking of the entitlement for services to the availability of resources, something that is seen by disability advocates as a denial of
an essential rights-based approach, creating dependence on the fiscal circumstances in play at any given time.

The definition of disability is a further bone of contention, and one that
raises fundamental questions. The Bill defines disability in terms of limitations
that arise as a result of 'an enduring physical, sensory, mental health or
intellectual impairment' – a definition clearly aimed at putting boundaries
around entitlements to services. In a social model of disability, however, the
thrust of sectoral plans and inclusive services is to minimise and even remove
the disabling impact of a society geared around 'able-bodied' norms. It seems
that the more successful that policy, the more people with disabilities may find
themselves undermining the case for the support services they may need to
retain their independence. Furthermore, how will people fare under this
legislation who experience short-term mental health problems or disabling
illnesses that have severe but not necessarily permanent impact, or people with
conditions such as epilepsy who, with the help of medication, can manage to
minimise but not necessarily remove all the consequences of the disability? In
this definition, then, we see the struggle between a welfare model of disability,
and a social model made manifest in a very explicit way.

Implementing a new policy focus

In drawing together conclusions based on the issues raised here, it is evident
that a sea change in disability policy in Ireland gained strong momentum in the
1990s and continued into the new century. Linked to this shift, parallel changes
began in the role of the health system in the lives of people with disabilities.
Within the health services, people with disabilities gained a direct voice in
regional service planning through the representation of the PwDI on the
regional co-ordinating committees of the health boards (in addition to the
representation for voluntary service providing organisations and the Disability
Federation of Ireland). It will be a continuing challenge for PwDI to put in
place mechanisms to ensure that local disabled people are genuinely empowered
and have gained influence. At the system level, changes have taken place in
structures and legislation which acknowledge that the needs of people with
disabilities are not exclusively the remit of the health services, and that the

disabled person, as citizen, has a claim on the policy and the resources of many other government departments and agencies.

Major areas of provision are now clearly acknowledged as being the remit of mainstream departments. The National Rehabilitation Board, which for over thirty years had responsibility for co-ordination of disability service and policy as well as provision of some key services, under the Department of Health and Children, was disbanded and its functions distributed across a range of mainstream departments and agencies including FÁS (the National Employment and Training Authority), the Department of Education and Science, and Comhairle, the body responsible for public information provision. The National Disability Authority, set up in 1999, whose remit is concerned with policy co-ordination, research, standard-setting and monitoring, operates under the auspices of the Department of Justice, Equality and Law Reform, thus giving structural focus to a new and healthy balance between the care agenda and the equality agenda.

As more pressure is brought to bear on other mainstream departments through the medium of sectoral plans to accept their responsibility for the inclusion of disabled citizens explicitly in their planning and budgeting, the remit of the health services will be to focus fully on essential personal support services as well as primary, secondary and tertiary health services. This emphasis in health service provision for people with physical disabilities is spelled out in the 2001 Health Strategy, *Quality and Fairness, A Health System for You,* Department of Health and Children (2001a), where the focus is on personal support services, support for carers, and a focus on quality and standards of service. These support services, care services and medical services will continue to have a very important role to play in securing independence, empowerment and a good quality of life for people with physical disabilities. The need for investment in these services is likely to continue to grow, as medical excellence expands the lifespan and quality of life of people with physical disabilities, and as their expectations for inclusion and participation, with the support of these services, also increases.

The shift away from a welfare perspective towards a rights-based model of public service provision for people with physical disabilities is now an integral part of philosophy and policy, even if the practice continues to evolve. The detailed implementation of practices such as information-giving and needs assessment will have a very powerful impact on the extent to which the philosophy moves to becoming embedded in the reality of the daily lived experience of people with disabilities. Undoubtedly there will continue to be an important place for caring local communities and peers who offer the kind of personal and mutual support which will always be beyond the capacity of the professional services providers in either the voluntary or state sector. The critical change, however, is likely to be an attitudinal change, through which all people with disabilities are acknowledged as equal participants in the planning, shaping and delivering of services, where they take responsibility for themselves as well as securing their rights and where a mutuality of respect informs all transactions and underpins decision making.

[See Editor's Addenda, chapter ii, p. 187]

Part 5

Lay health beliefs and practices

Chapter 13

Breastfeeding: issues in the implementation of policy

Aoife Rickard

There is a widespread popular perception – supported by much factual evidence – that rates of breastfeeding in the Republic of Ireland compare unfavourably with other countries, both in terms of the proportion of mothers who start to breastfeed and how long they continue. It has frequently been noted in the press that Ireland's breastfeeding rates are low by international standards, and lowest among the lowest socio-economic groups. This may appear paradoxical, given the fact that Ireland had achieved some of the highest standards of perinatal health care in the EU and is 'rated among the best countries in the world in caring for young children' (*The Irish Times*, 8 April 1992). The same article in *The Irish Times* pointed out that Ireland's children are cherished, defended and safeguarded, and that the decline in the figures for breastfeeding is 'one exception to Ireland's exemplary treatment of its children'. The decline had happened in spite of efforts to promote breastfeeding from the 1970s by a number of agencies, and especially by the Department of Health which launched a National Breastfeeding Policy in 1994 to protect and support breastfeeding. Secondly, Ireland has a low rate of female participation in the labour force: in 1980 only 29.7 of all women, including married women, participated in the labour force compared with Britain, France and Germany, where the figures were respectively 62.3, 57.0, and 56.2 (see table 13.1). One might expect that mothers remaining at home would be more likely to breastfeed, and that the rate in Ireland should therefore be higher rather than lower in consequence. Why then has Ireland not succeeded in raising the numbers of women breastfeeding?

Table 13.1 **Female participation in the labour force, 1980**

	Married Women (%)	All women, including married (%)
Ireland	16.7	29.7
France	52.6	57.0
Germany	54.4	56.2
United Kingdom	57.2	62.3

Source: Callan and Farrell (1991).

These figures are for 1980 – now out of date – but relevant to a 1982 survey, which is still the most comprehensive study of breastfeeding in Ireland. It is certainly not for any lack of public awareness of the problem. In order to document the extent of public concern and the public's perception of the problem, I analysed all the references to breastfeeding in *The Irish Times* from 1992 to 1996. Two main points emerged:

- that in recent years there have been fairly frequent articles bemoaning low breastfeeding rates and speculating about the reasons for them
- that there is very little hard data: public comment has been based almost wholly on the findings of one major study in 1982, and neither the Central Statistics Office nor the hospitals have kept records until the last few years.

Ireland today in comparative perspective

To see just how low Ireland's rates of breastfeeding are, one must place the country in a comparative context. Ireland, whose rate at three months of approximately 15 per cent (Hurley, 1994: 14), is almost half that of the United Kingdom, a country whose breastfeeding rates are not particularly high either. Table 13.2 shows how rates are highest among the countries of the periphery within the world-system, and lowest among the countries of the core.

One can see from this table how unfavourably Ireland stands. The prevalence of breastfeeding is remarkably higher at three months in the UK and USA than in Ireland. For the 1981 national survey reported by McSweeney and Kevany (1982), *Infant Feeding Practices in Ireland,* information was obtained on 1,195 mothers, and the national distribution by feeding methods on discharge from hospital are given in table 13.3. It can be seen from table 13.3 that on discharge from hospital only 32 per cent of mothers were breastfeeding. This also corresponds with the figures from the Department of Health's Perinatal Statistics Reports, 1985–93 (see table 13.4).

Table 13.2 **Prevalence of breastfeeding in selected countries: Percentage of mothers breastfeeding 1980–8**

Position/Country Periphery	3 months %	6 months %	12 months %
Tanzania	100	90	70
Ethiopia	—	97	95
Nepal	92	92	82
Bangladesh	91	86	82
Kenya	96	82	67
Sri Lanka	95	81	68
Senegal	94	94	82
Cameroon	92	90	77
Semi-periphery			
Indonesia	98	97	76
Egypt	90	87	81
Ecuador	86	74	48
Thailand	83	79	68
Chile	81	57	20
Semi-core			
China	66	58	34
Brazil	66	58	34
South Korea	58	40	27
Core			
United Kingdom	26	22	—
Canada	53	30	—
United States	33	24	—
Japan	72	52	—

Source: Adapted from Macintosh (1996).

Table 13.3 **Methods of feeding on discharge from hospital**

	%
Breast only	29
Breast and complementary	2
Breast and supplementary	1
Bottle only	68

Source: McSweeney and Kevany, (1982: 15).

Table 13.4 **Percentage of mothers breastfeeding on discharge from hospital**

1985	1986	1987	1988	1989	1990	1991	1993
34.1	33.9	33.2	32.3	32.8	31.8	31.9	33.9

Source: Department of Health Perinatal Statistics Reports, several.

The findings from the McSweeney and Kevany survey (1982) revealed:

- That women who breastfeed are likely to be older when giving birth than those who bottle-feed.

- Breastfeeders are from a higher socio-economic group.

- Breastfeeders have also been found to have a higher level of educational achievement than bottle-feeders.

- The closer the proximity mothers live to their families of origin the more likely they are to be bottle-fed.

Well over half the sample were found to have decided on feeding method before pregnancy. A number of factors which influenced their choice emerged from this and other studies. Roughly in reverse chronological order, they included:

Return to Work. An Irish national survey in 1986 found that a quarter of women said their duration of breastfeeding was decided by their return to work (Hurley, 1994: 49). What is interesting to find is that Norway, the country with the highest incidence and prevalence of breastfeeding, has very extensive structural supports for breastfeeding mothers. These supports include maternity leave having been extended from 12 weeks in the early 1970s to 46 weeks in 1993 for women who have been in employment for six of the ten weeks prior to giving birth and a two-hour nursing break a day for working mothers (Hurley, 1994: 49). The structural constraints in Ireland may be a factor affecting Irelands breastfeeding rates especially when one looks at Norway's structural supports and high rates of breastfeeding.

Hospital Experience. According to an article in *The Irish Times* (21 February 1994), the low incidence of breastfeeding among Irish women may be directly attributed to the conflicting advice women receive from health care professionals and family and friends. Also, a considerable proportion of Irish mothers who are breastfeeding on discharge discontinue during the early weeks. Many mothers also expressed demand for more information and help on returning home from hospital. Unlike in the UK, where there are publicly funded community-based midwives who visit the mother every day for the first ten days after the baby is born, in Ireland there is no such extensive back-up service (*The Irish Times*, 4 March 1994).

Husbands' attitudes. The 1982 survey also took into account husbands' attitudes towards breastfeeding. This survey and studies in other countries have found that husbands influence the decision and there is also evidence that a husband's support for breastfeeding is associated with its duration (Hurley, 1994). Connolly et al. (1998) found young men's attitudes were positive towards breastfeeding. They believed this was something girls should be aware of before initiating pregnancy, as it is seen to be a supportive factor rather than an inhibiting one.

Wider network of friends. There is also evidence of a connection between breastfeeding and having a wide network of friends. In the 1982 survey it was found that 63.5 per cent of mothers who bottle-fed, but only 40 per cent of the breastfeeders, said that the majority of their acquaintances were bottle-feeders. Conversely, 16 per cent of bottle-feeders and 37.5 per cent of breastfeeders reported that the majority of their acquaintances were breastfeeders (McSweeney and Kevany, 1982: 32).

Mothers' influence. An interesting factor influencing mothers' choice of feeding is family and friends with whom the mother is in regular contact. More of the breastfeeders than the women who bottle-fed were actually breastfed themselves. This clearly points out that mothers have a very strong influence over their daughters' choice of feeding method. In Ireland, however, breast-feeding had skipped a generation, so that the mothers who are influencing their daughters now were more than likely to have bottle-fed and this is one of the reasons why Ireland's breastfeeding rates are not increasing.

Embarrassment. According to McSweeney and Kevany (1982: 35), embarrassment about breastfeeding is a handicap in a society where rates of breastfeeding have fallen so low and where the breast as a sex symbol has been emphasised so much that it can be seen as immodest and unnatural, and even immoral to breastfeed. Sixteen years later, Connolly et al. (1998) still found embarrassment and discomfort to be the most prevalent emotions expressed in relation to the subject of breastfeeding, with the majority of their respondents (teenagers of both sexes still in school) disapproving of breastfeeding in public. In a study by Wiley and Merriman (1996), one in four women mentioned embarrassment as the reason they chose not to breastfeed. The 1982 survey also showed that 10 per cent of those who bottle-fed specifically mentioned the reason they chose to bottle-feed was due to embarrassment about breastfeeding. A survey in the UK during the 1980s showed 11 per cent of bottle-feeders mentioning embarrassment as the reason they did not breastfeed (Hurley, 1994: 47). McSweeney and Kevany asked both breastfeeding and bottle-feeding mothers whether they would mind breastfeeding in various situations; the two groups varied quite clearly in their levels of embarrassment regarding breast-feeding. A surprising 9.5 per cent of bottle-feeders said they would be embarrassed to breastfeed in front of their husbands. Thirty-nine per cent of the women from this group said they would be embarrassed to breastfeed in front of their mothers and 80 per cent would be embarrassed in front of their fathers (1982: 30). Embarrassment rates for breastfeeders were lower, but they were found to be substantial in some situations. In all cases a higher percentage of women from the manual than from the non-manual groups were embarrassed about breastfeeding in the various situations. This can be linked to a higher percentage of breastfeeders among the non-manual group, indicating that, as the occurrence of breastfeeding increases, levels of embarrassment decrease because many breastfeeding mothers expressed the feeling that their inhibition was more in response to anticipated embarrassment of others than actual embarrassment on their own part (McSweeney and Kevany, 1982). Connolly et al. (1998: 89) believe the source of this embarrassment and discomfort was due to 'looking at the naked breast and its exposure, accompanied by confusion around the dual feeding/sexual role of the female breast'.

Long-term trends in Western Europe

Several of the explanations offered for low rates of breastfeeding in Ireland, such as the influence of earlier generations, of husbands and of social networks, and especially the role of embarrassment, give us a hint that attitudes may be deeply rooted in the past, and thus not very easy to change in the short term. One needs to examine longer trends through history in order to show how we have arrived at the situation today. There is limited historical evidence in relation to Ireland, but what there is suggests that, although rates of breastfeeding are low here today, the long-term pattern of change in child-rearing and feeding has been broadly similar in most Western European countries. So I shall draw on evidence from other countries to reconstruct the long-term general trends.

From historical evidence the decline in rates of breastfeeding has been identified by many as occurring in the mid-nineteenth century as a result of rapid industrialisation and the rise of the 'scientific' (usually male) experts in childbirth and to the expansion of the baby milk industry. It seems, however, that longer-term processes have had and still have an effect on women's decisions to breastfeed. These influences are deep-rooted and have been developing over time. I hope to uncover the 'problem' as having a much longer history and show that changes in underlying attitudes towards breastfeeding started before technological advances.

Throughout most of pre-industrial Europe maternal breastfeeding was seen as the normal and most superior method of infant feeding (Fildes, 1986). But non-maternal breastfeeding, commonly known as wet-nursing, has been recorded since ancient times. In France, going back to the thirteenth century, royal children were fed by wet-nurses; and at social levels below the royal line evidence of wet-nursing goes back to the Middle Ages. During the eighteenth century the wet-nurses were usually peasant women who took the babies from the cities to the rural cottages for the nursing period. By the nineteenth century it was preferred to recruit rural women as live-in nurses. During the seventeenth and eighteenth century wet-nursing reached its peak in England although it was never as widespread as it was in other parts of Europe, especially in France, where Sussman (1982) points out that in the two centuries from 1715 to 1914 wet-nurses were used by urban artisans and shopkeepers and not just by the well-to-do. Whatever detailed national differences there might have been, during the seventeenth century the reliance on wet-nurses by the upper classes was widespread across Europe. MacCurtain and O'Dowd (1991: 276) noted that even in Ireland, 'those [babies] of the wealthy were consigned almost entirely to the care of wet-nurses and servants'. Why was it that women from the upper classes did not breastfeed? Palmer (1988) says it was not due to their participation in public life, nor to do with the fact that suckling in public was not accepted, for at that time it was. There are several possible explanations. One important consideration is that employing a wet nurse was – at first for upper-class women, and subsequently for many middle-class mothers too – a sign of social distinction, in spite of medical opinion consistently recommending breastfeeding. Later, however, there are signs that wet-nurses were drawn less from lower strata than before, that they came to be seen as a potential source of disease, especially syphilis, and more especially of social contamination. In short, wet-nursing ceased to be respectable and ceased to be a mark of distinction. By the nineteenth century, the decline of wet-nursing added impetus to the search for safe and effective methods of artificial feeding.

Breastfeeding and civilising processes

I now want to deal with changing attitudes towards the body, such as feelings of shame and embarrassment, and how these affected changing attitudes towards breastfeeding. It is these more deep-rooted meanings affecting people's behaviour which leads me on to examining Elias's account of the civilising of the body, which historically shows how attitudes to the body form over time.

Elias (1994) examines how particular forms of behaviour came to be defined as 'good' and 'bad', 'appropriate' and 'inappropriate' and so on. He argues that the change came about through structural transformation in society which occurred very slowly, bringing with it a compulsion to check one's behaviour. Elias depicts not only changes in surface manners but changes in people's feelings and attitudes towards the body – the psychological changes that underlay the outward changes. Although he does not himself discuss breastfeeding, his explanations appear by extension to be directly relevant to why rates of breast-feeding have declined. He takes the late Middle Ages as a convenient starting point, as it was during this period that a distinct acceleration is evident in the pace at which the social standards of behaviour and attitudes to the body change. Changes in relation to infant feeding patterns became noticeable around this time, though at first they affected limited sections of society. Breastfeeding was carried out by the majority of women simply as the only means of feeding the baby and as another task to be done. There seem not to have been any problems related to it, nor negative attitudes towards women's bodies as there are today. The change he describes seems also to apply quite precisely in relation to breastfeeding, as it is obvious that fewer women came to breastfeed, and that the reasons put forward as to why this was so do not adequately explain the low rates. There seems to be something more deep-rooted and it is precisely this which Elias uncovers and which holds true to women's reluctance to breastfeed.

Elias traces changes in many aspects of manners and habitus (deeply incul-cated unconscious ways of acting and behaving) from about the time of the Renaissance to social conduct in general – the compulsion to check one's behaviour increased and the threshold of shame and embarrassment advanced. This coincided with a move towards wet-nursing, as the women of the upper classes in general no longer wanted to be seen breastfeeding their own children.

Within court societies, highly detailed codes of body management were institutionalised to differentiate people on the basis of their worth. This in turn heightened people's tendency to observe their own bodily behaviour and that of others. It became necessary for court people to develop 'an extraordinarily sensitive feeling for the status and importance that should be attributed to a person in society on the basis of his bearing, speech, manner or appearance' (Shilling, 1993: 155). This may be connected with why it was at this time that wet-nursing reached its peak in Britain and France. Upper-class women were not to be seen breastfeeding their infants but instead to be sitting in ornamental idleness. Some of the other general changes which occurred at this time and continued throughout the centuries were the rationalisation of sleeping cycles, stricter taboos concerning where to sleep, and sexuality being moved to the more private areas. 'The movement towards things no longer being spoken about ran in conjunction with a movement towards moving many of the same things behind the scenes of social life' (Mennell, 1998: 43).

Elias focused on the most basic, 'natural' or 'animalistic' of human functions – eating, drinking, defecating, sleeping, blowing one's nose – because these are the things that humans cannot biologically avoid doing, no matter what culture or age they live in (Mennell, 1998: 36), so that when change occurs in the social standards governing them, it is particularly easy to observe.

Breastfeeding belongs to this category of 'natural' human functions. All of these functions, and more, were increasingly hedged around with rules and restrictions, and many were moved behind the scenes of social life. The bedroom became one of the most 'private' and 'intimate' areas of human life. Although it may now be regarded as unacceptable to compare breastfeeding with these other functions, it is quite apparent that greater care was taken regarding the company in which breastfeeding was carried out (or more often not). 'The hiding behind the scenes of what has become distasteful is one of the most characteristic features of the civilising process in Europe' (Mennell, 1998: 43). So we can already see evidence of breastfeeding becoming 'distasteful' as it moves to more private arenas; in turn there began a decline in breastfeeding, which continued in tandem with heightening social standards of self-constraint and changing manners in relation to the body.

Reasons for the change

Having outlined some of the characteristics involved in the development of the civilising process in relation to the 'civilised body', such as the progressive refinement of manners, the advance of thresholds of shame and embarrassment, the hiding behind the scenes of social life functions which have become embarrassing, and the psychological changes which accompanied these processes, it is necessary to identify the major factors which contributed to these changes and set them in motion.

Material Reasons

Can the decline of breastfeeding be related simply to technological advances? Did breastfeeding persist because of the lack of scientific and technological knowledge – because the bottle and formula milk had not been invented? The answer is simply no – these reasons do not supply an adequate answer, because attitudes towards the natural functions began to change before the invention of the knife and fork, the toilet or the bottle. Attitudes towards the body were changing and moving behind the scenes before the widespread use of the bottle. Women who breastfed were doing so in private, and more and more women of the upper classes were employing wet-nurses.

Reasons of health and hygiene

Surely considerations of hygiene played an important part especially in the Middle Ages when the lack of medical expertise and the spread of infectious diseases were widespread. Elias (1994: 93–5) says that medical justifications would have played only a minor role in bringing about higher standards but this could not have caused these developments because once again it was only after manners had changed that these functions came to be seen as unhealthy and socially unacceptable. The fear of syphilis spread among mothers whose babies were being wet-nursed when the class of wet-nurses had already begun to change. It was a different class of wet-nurses about which this fear arose. They were no longer respectable rural women but were young inexperienced girls (sometimes prostitutes) who in some cases had abandoned their own babies in order to make a living out of wet-nursing. There was now a much greater demand for an alternative feeding method, and pressure from the upper classes was brought to bear on the medical experts to develop an artificial and safer alternative. Shame and fear accompany certain forms of behaviour which would have been absent previously and these feelings gradually spread from the standard setting circles to larger circles. Once such feelings arise and become firmly established in society they tend to be reproduced as long as the structure of social relations is not changed dramatically.

Reasons of respect

So what other reasons were given for this change in 'proper' and 'improper', 'socially acceptable' and 'socially unacceptable' ways of behaving? The reasons most often given in manners books from the sixteenth to the eighteenth centuries to justify new standards which came about were that behaviour in the past was relatively unrestrained and showed lack of respect towards social superiors. An illustration of this is given by Elias in relation to exposure of the body. At first it became offensive and distasteful to expose oneself in any way to those of higher social rank. Later, especially by the nineteenth century, shame was felt equally by superiors in the presence of inferiors – the social command not to show oneself naked applied to everyone equally. It became imprinted in the child as the natural way to behave. As bodily exposure became less 'normal' in society, so natural bodily functions came to be carried out in private. This behaviour became an automatic, unconscious self-restraint among both children and adults. What Mennell (1998: 47) terms 'reasons of respect' are clues to the beginnings of Elias's explanation of the dynamic of the civilising process. It is a process which consists in important respects of changing ways of showing and demanding respect which occurs because of the changes in structures in social relations. The main cause for the changes which were occurring according to Shilling (1993) concerned the search for distinction in the context of more intensive social competition for the ascent through the ranks of society. For example, this process could possibly be seen in relation to infant feeding. The upper classes distinguished themselves as an elite by sending their children to be wet-nursed; when this method trickled down and was imitated by the middle classes, the upper-classes searched for a different way to feed their children, in order to retain their eliteness. They turned to their doctors for a different feeding method and artificial feeding became popular among this group, not because it was necessarily better for the child, but it was a different method from those used by lower classes and it showed that these families had money and access to doctors for expert advice.

Breastfeeding and informalising processes

Elias's theory of civilising processes helps to show why a decline in breast-feeding came about and continued until very recent decades. Yet in many countries in recent years, rates of breastfeeding have begun to rise. That upturn appears to run parallel with the apparent reversal of many of the trends in other aspects of manners which Elias depicted in *The Civilising Process* – a reversal which has led to debates about contemporary 'informalising processes' and the 'permissive society'. In contrast, rates of breastfeeding in Ireland remain low and there is little evidence of them as yet rising in line with the international trend. We are therefore left with not a single but a dual problem: we still have to attempt to explain why Irish rates of breastfeeding are so low, but also why elsewhere they are rising.

Informalising processes

The 1960s and 1970s are often regarded in many countries as a time when there occurred an increase in 'permissiveness', with a relaxation of morals and codes of conduct and a pervasive informalisation of social behaviour. Many modes of conduct that were formerly forbidden were now allowed, particularly in relation to sexual matters (Wouters, 1986). This is how the young people differentiated their behaviour from that of their parents. They did not see themselves as just rejecting their parents' social code of conduct, but all social codes; they saw themselves as simply able to choose, as individuals. They did not have to follow any social code and argued that nobody should follow codes imposed by society, instead they should 'conduct their behaviour in accordance with their own individuality and in accordance with what they sense that others as individuals want or need' (Wouters, 1977: 440). Part of this current was an explicit wish to get 'back to nature', manifested in (among many other things) young mothers carrying their babies in slings and breastfeeding them.

But Wouters has argued that this perception of informalising processes was highly misleading. He has argued that 'a highly controlled decontrolling of emotional controls' was at the root of the informalisation process (Mennell, 1998: 243), which he illustrated by giving the example of changing power rela-tions between parents and children. He showed how internal standards of conduct between parents and children required less use of external constraints (*Fremdzwänge*) and more use of self-constraints (*Selbstzwänge*) especially among children (Wouters, 1986) and therefore a continuation of the main thrust of the civilising process. Wouters tells us that many modes of conduct which were formerly forbidden are now permitted, particularly in relation to sexual matters, but that this depends on a higher degree of internalisation of mutually expected self-constraints. It is easier for people consciously to think and speak about sexual matters, and both to express and to restrain their sexuality than it was for the Victorian generations. How does this relate to breastfeeding in Ireland?

The special case of Ireland?

The onset of these processes in Ireland seems to have been later than elsewhere. Religion, especially in Ireland where people have been very devout, has – as we shall see – had an effect on how people perceive their bodies and on attitudes and beliefs in society in general, such as man as breadwinner, woman as home maker. Irish people have followed very closely the teachings of the Catholic Church. The change which Wouters has shown to have occurred in other societies can be seen to be occurring in relation to religion in Ireland today among the younger generations. It may have an effect in bringing about a change in attitudes towards the body, and (as I shall argue) that may in turn bring about an increase in rates of breastfeeding.

Post-famine Ireland marked the rise in the hegemony of the Catholic priest. What is peculiar to Ireland, and had a lasting effect, is that the civilising process took place in and through the Catholic Church (Inglis, 1987). As the Catholic Church was the most respected institution in Ireland and remained so for longer than elsewhere in Europe, this can be seen to be a reason why Irish people are so ashamed of their bodies and why breastfeeding in Ireland is uncommon. The civilising process transformed open, passionate bodies into closed, moral bodies (Inglis, 1987). In Ireland it was through priests, brothers and nuns that these transformations were inculcated in the Irish people. The church sought to instil in people feelings of shame and guilt about the body. Irish Catholicism is marked by its private nature.

Inglis (1987) notes how the priest and the church acted as a civilising agents in Irish society and used mechanisms to moralise and civilise the body. It was through the beliefs in the church that people first learned to control their bodies. The Catholic Church managed very successfully to instil this way of thinking, living and acting in the Irish people through various means. Through pastoral visitation and confession the priest began to supervise all aspects of social life. Priests acted as what Blanshard (1954: 155) called 'moral policemen'. Many stories have been told about priests supervising dances and separating partners for dancing too close to one another. Since the practice of the Catholic religion in Ireland was viewed as a way of distinguishing oneself from the Protestant and English way of life and as a means of gaining status, the fear of condemnation by priests was great. The success of adhering to rules of the church depended greatly on regular attendance at confession. It was through confession that the Church managed to control the sexual lives of the Irish people, especially women and young girls. 'Confession played a crucial role in sexualising the body' (Inglis 1987: 149). During confession, activities of the body were examined and suitable penances administered. Through a thorough investigation of the penitent's sexual practices a sense of private guilt and public shame was experienced. It was through such an examination procedure that 'ignorant savages' were made to feel self-conscious about their bodies and thereby became constituted as moral human beings (Inglis, 1987: 149).

If these feelings about the body were instilled in the Irish people through the Catholic Church it comes as no surprise as to why rates of breastfeeding in Ireland are so low. Many women would have been made feel ashamed to breast-feed their children, not only in public but in private as well. As Elias (1994: 492ff) says, these feelings become so strong and inculcated within oneself, that they are experienced even when one is alone.

Controlling sex as a practice and a discourse, argues Inglis (1987), became one of the main strategies by which the Catholic Church maintained its power. The 1960s saw a new awareness of and discourse about sexuality. This occurred mainly via an overspill from British television transmitters enabling people along the east coast to pick up BBC and ITV. Although there was a new sexualisation of the Irish body around the late 1960s, the ability to discuss these changes in social and cultural practices did not come about until the 1980s. It would appear that the process of informalisation, like the civilising process, has been slow to occur in Ireland but that we are beginning to see its effects. Whelan (1994), comparing European and Irish values, finds Irish values on matters like abortion and sexual freedom to be distinctly conservative. Whelan is not convinced that the Catholic Church in Ireland has undergone major change but 'has remained insulated from secularisation influences' (1994: 43). As it relates specifically to younger cohorts of Irish people, however, Whelan's evidence seems to show that after a time lag of some decades Irish Catholics are following western norms. This has occurred around the time that the moral monopoly of the Catholic Church in Ireland began markedly to break down. But, as we have seen, feelings of shame and unease in relation to the body have formed only slowly in the course of long-term social processes, and it is equally true that they could not disappear overnight. This would help to explain why informalisation or the so-called 'permissive society' came late to Ireland.

Chapter 14

Health, illness and lifestyles

Desmond McCluskey

According to the World Health Organisation (1986), the first 60 years or so of the twentieth century could be termed the 'medical era', in which the dominant approach to health care was based on mass vaccination and the extensive use of antibiotics. Now, industrialised countries have entered upon a 'post-medical era' in which physical well-being is undermined by certain types of individual behaviour (for example, smoking), failures of social organisation (loneliness), economic factors (poverty, overeating) and factors in the physical environment (pollution), that are not amenable to improvement by medicine, which today has only a limited capacity to effect further improvements in health. The WHO goes on to suggest that, while in the medical era health policy has been concerned mainly with how medical care is to be provided and paid for, in the new post-medical era it will focus on the attainment of good health and well-being. At first, changes in individual lifestyles were seen as the key means to achieve this goal. Subsequently, attention has been directed more and more at the influence on health of economic, social and ecological factors. In spite of this, control over personal behaviour is still accorded a major role.

In their analyses of health and illness behaviours, sociologists have employed both micro and macro approaches. From a micro or individualistic perspective, behavioural differences are explained in terms of personal characteristics and individual motivations and experiences. From a macro or structural perspective, variations in behaviour are seen as arising from social and cultural forces, including the influence of such factors as gender, age, socio-economic status, educational attainment, religion, race and ethnicity.

Micro approach

Various socio-psychological models have been developed to explain health and/ or illness behaviour (see Becker and Maiman, 1983). Though, generally, these accounts emphasise an individualistic approach many also incorporate structural influences in their formulations. Two models in which the individualistic perspective predominates and which have been widely utilised are the Health Belief Model (HBM) and Health Locus of Control (HLC) scales.

The HBM, originally formulated by Rosenstock (1966), proposes that people will take action to prevent illness or to restore health if they feel (i) susceptible to a particular disease; (ii) that contracting the disease would have serious consequences, organic or social; (iii) that taking a specific action will be effective in reducing the threat or in minimising the consequences if the disease is contracted; (iv) that the benefits involved in the proposed action outweigh any costs, physical, financial or social that might be incurred; and finally (v) a cue to action is often needed to trigger the appropriate behaviour – this cue can be either internal, for example symptoms, or external such as advice from others or mass media communications. A general concern about health matters was included as an additional motivating factor in subsequent versions of the model (see Becker, 1979). These later formulations also included the influence of sociodemographic and personality variables. The HBM has provided a useful framework for investigating health, illness and sick role behaviours (Becker, 1979) and has been employed successfully in studies of preventive health practices and adherence to medically prescribed behaviours (Ogden, 1996; Cockerham, 1998). However, the model has been criticised on a number of counts: (1) though helpful in examining disease specific behaviours it is less applicable to understanding preventive health actions in general (Weiss and Lonnquist, 1999); (2) the operationalisation of its conceptual components presents considerable problems (Sheeran and Abraham, 1996); and (3) though specific components have been shown to be associated with differences in behaviour, when taken together they often explain only a small amount of the variance in compliance behaviour (Morgan et al., 1985).

A Health Locus of Control (HLC) scale was originally developed by Wallston et al. (1976) as a unidimensional measure of people's beliefs that their health is or is not determined by their own behaviour. On one end of the scale are the 'health internals', those who believe that one stays or becomes healthy or sick as a result of one's own behaviour. On the other end are the 'health externals', those who take the view that one's health is determined by such things as luck, fate or chance, factors over which they have little control. Subsequently, Wallston and Wallston (1978) developed a Multidimensional Health Locus of Control (MHLC) scale which incorporated the influence of powerful others, for example, doctors, as an added external dimension. Cockerham (1998) suggests that locus of control measures have proved useful in analysing both health and illness behaviour. He cites the work of Seeman and Seeman (1983) who found that a low sense of internal control could be significantly associated with less self-initiated preventive care, less optimism about the effectiveness of early treatment, poorer self-rated health, more illness and bed confinement and greater dependence on doctors. On the other hand,

Norman and Bennett (1996) argue that the role of health control scales in predicting behaviour is weak since the amount of variance explained by the construct is low.

Macro approach

Weiss and Lonnquist (1999) draw attention to studies in the United States and Britain which point clearly to an association between social factors and *health* behaviour. For example, it was found that women were more likely than men to wear car seat belts, but less likely to smoke cigarettes and to be heavy drinkers; men, on the other hand, were more likely to get adequate physical exercise. It emerged, too, that health behaviour was associated with social class, level of education, occupation and income: people with lower levels of education, those in manual occupations, and those with lower incomes were more likely to smoke cigarettes but less likely to take physical exercise. Cockerham (1998), however, argues that studies in the United States, Germany and other European countries found considerable similarities in health lifestyles across social classes. At the same time, he observes that those of lower socio-economic status are much less likely than others to use preventive health services such as medical and dental check-ups. He notes, too, that smoking is more common among those with lower levels of education and income. Whitehead (1992) also records that there is plenty of evidence from British studies that members of lower occupational classes make less use of preventive services for themselves and their children.

Variations in *illness* behaviour are also found to be related to social factors. Cockerham (1998) refers to numerous studies that indicate that, when ill, women are more likely to utilise medical services than men and the elderly are more likely to do so than young and middle-aged adults. Cockerham also cites evidence that people in lower income groups have higher utilisation rates than those in middle and upper income categories. However, he points out that, when actual *need* for health services is taken into account, lower income persons appear to use fewer services relative to their needs. A British study by Blaxter (1984) concluded that the higher consultation rates with doctors for lower occupational groups were justified by the more severe nature of the symptoms they experienced. Other findings suggest that the use of health services is influenced by what Freidson (1970) calls the *lay referral system*: potential patients usually discuss their symptoms with a significant other, most frequently a family member, before deciding to seek professional help (McKinlay, 1973; Scambler et al., 1981).

A striking example of the macro approach to illness behaviour is Zola's study of patients attending three Boston clinics (Zola, 1966). The study focused on the role of cultural factors in explaining differential responses to what were essentially similar disease conditions of the eye, ear, nose or throat. When Zola compared the responses of Irish-American and Italian-American patients it emerged that for the same diagnosis the Italians expressed and complained of more symptoms, more bodily areas affected, and more kinds of dysfunction than did the Irish, and more often felt that their symptoms affected their interpersonal behaviour. The Irish tended to understate their symptoms and to deny that pain was a feature of their experience.

In theorising about the interplay of culture and symptoms Zola suggests that Italian and Irish ways of communicating illness reflect different coping mechanisms and preferred ways of handling problems within their divergent cultures. For the Italians the overstatement of symptoms is a form of defence mechanism called *dramatisation.* Dramatisation seems to cope with anxiety by repeatedly over-expressing it and in this way dissipating it. This, according to Zola, reflects the common Italian flair for show and spectacle which, it is said, helps cover up omnipresent tragedy and hardship and makes daily life more bearable. But, argues Zola, if the Italian view of life is expressed through its fiestas, for the Irish it is expressed through its fasts. Historically, life for the Irish was marked by lengthy periods of deprivation and the postponement of sexual gratification and marriage. If life was black and long-suffering the less said the better. For the Irish the response of *denial* and underplaying of symptoms seems to represent a culturally prescribed and supported defence mechanism appropriate for their psychological and physical survival. While the validity of Zola's explanation of these differential responses to symptoms is open to question, the study remains important in that it shows how variations in socio-cultural background may lead to different definitions and responses to essentially the same illness condition.

Health and illness behaviour in Ireland

The present chapter is based on the findings of a study of the health beliefs and practices of lay people in Ireland by McCluskey (1989). This has been the only large quantitative study carried out in the Republic of Ireland employing a sociological perspective and analysed within a sociological and socio-psycho-logical framework. Two other important surveys have been conducted more recently of the health actions of lay people in Ireland, based on large national samples (see Friel et al., 1999; Centre for Health Promotion Studies, 2003). But though these have provided a wide range of information on people's health behaviour, the findings have not been analysed from a sociological perspective, employing sociological concepts and theories and drawing on sociological literature. (It is worth noting that the findings of these two studies are consistent with those of McCluskey.) The objectives of the McCluskey study were to discover how lay people in general conceive of health and illness and what actions they take to promote good health or to remedy illness. Using a largely structured questionnaire, interviews were conducted with 475 people, randomly selected in two locations, Dublin city and a rural area in another Leinster county. The findings of the survey, in so far as they relate to the definitions and perceived causes of health and illness, have been further elaborated by the author (McCluskey, 1997). The account which follows gives a fuller treatment of the second half of the study: the health and illness behaviour of the study population.

Micro approach to the data

In the presentation of the main findings a micro approach is adopted at first, with variations in behaviour analysed in terms of the personal characteristics of the respondents and their health and illness experiences. Subsequently, a macro approach is employed when their health and illness behaviours are examined in relation to socio-demographic variables.

Health Behaviour

The terms 'health behaviour' and 'preventive health behaviour' are often used interchangeably to denote the actions people take to promote good health or to avoid illness. The distinction has been made between *primary* prevention where the objective is to avoid disease or injury altogether, *secondary* prevention which aims at catching the disease or injury in its early stages before any real damage has occurred, and *tertiary* prevention which is concerned with minimising deterioration in an ill person and maximising recovery. Health behaviour, as the term is generally used, tends to focus on primary and secondary prevention. However, it embraces a wide range of behaviours, all of which it is difficult to accommodate within a single definition. It includes such varied actions as taking physical exercise, avoiding certain foods, refraining from smoking, having medical or dental check-ups, being immunised against disease, wearing a car seat-belt and observing safety regulations at work.

It is important to point out that the study presented here was concerned with self-defined health behaviour, that is, actions which people perceive as conducive to good health, whether such actions are medically approved of or not and whether they are objectively effective or not. Two new terms were introduced in the study: manifest health behaviour and latent health behaviour. One can distinguish between those behaviours which people engage in with the specific intention of promoting or maintaining their health – *manifest health behaviour*, and those which they perform without such a conscious decision even though, at the same time, they may perceive them as health-protective – *latent health behaviour.* Latent health behaviour, as the term is used here, does not imply that people are unaware of the health consequences of their actions, only that the actions have not as their primary or conscious objective the promoting of one's health.

The respondents were asked in open-ended questions what they did or avoided in the interests of their health. Their answers were taken to represent their manifest health behaviour – the actions they took with the specific intention of promoting or protecting their health. The overwhelming majority of the respondents (77 per cent) indicated that they engaged in at least one form of health behaviour (table 14.1). In general their manifest health behaviour reflected their perceptions of the causes of health and illness (see McCluskey, 1989; 1997). Since food was the factor most commonly perceived as affecting health, it was, therefore, not surprising that the most frequently mentioned health practice focused on food: eating what was considered healthy food and avoiding what was regarded as unhealthy food. So too, references to physical exercise, not smoking and getting sufficient rest reflected other perceived causes of good health. There was also reference to taking care of oneself, including keeping warm and avoiding getting wet.

Table 14.1 **Health behaviour of respondents**

Health behaviour	Percentage respondents*
Eating healthy food, avoiding fatty or unhealthy food	29.9
Exercising physically, keeping fit	25.5
Taking care of oneself, keeping warm, avoiding getting wet	20.4
Not smoking	15.2
Getting sufficient rest or sleep, avoiding late nights or overwork	14.5
Eating moderately, keeping weight in check	8.4
Not drinking	7.4
Other forms of health behaviour	33.1
Did not engage in any form of health behaviour	22.7
N	**475**

*Percentages sum to more than 100 because some respondents engaged in more than one form of health behaviour.
Source: McCluskey (1989).

It must be remembered that what is being discussed here is behaviour performed with the primary intention of protecting or promoting one's health, that is, *manifest* health behaviour. Hence, though very large proportions of the respondents indicated that they did not smoke cigarettes or that they regularly took physical exercise (see below) very many did not include these among their manifest health behaviours.

The findings of an American study (Harris and Guten, 1979) indicate that virtually everyone performs some health protective behaviours but the most commonly performed activities do not include use of the health services. A similar picture emerged from the study being discussed here. The respondents were presented with two lists of health measures and were asked to specify how frequently they performed each measure listed. The first list involved contact with health care professionals, the second list referred to behaviours where such contacts were not involved. On the first list the respondents were asked, 'Even when there is nothing wrong with you how frequently do you do the following: (i) visit a doctor for a medical check-up; (ii) visit a dentist for a dental check-up?'

Visits to a doctor or dentist for check-ups were infrequent occurrences for the majority of the respondents. Only 28 per cent indicated that they sought a medical check-up at least once a year and an even smaller proportion (25 per cent) had a dental check-up at least once annually. Moreover, it was not established whether having a medical check-up was entirely voluntary; many may have been required by their employer or by the nature of their work to take such action. This may help to explain why the proportion reporting to have done so (28 per cent) was considerably greater than the proportion making a similar claim (8 per cent) in another Irish study (Tussing, 1985). What is clear is that a regular medical examination did not appear a top priority with most members in the sample population.

Table 14.2 **Frequency of participation in specific health behaviours**

	Always	Most of the time	Less frequently	Rarely/ never	N
	%	%	%	%	%
Wearing a car seat-belt*	46.2	17.5	12.3	34.0	474
Sufficient exercise	36.4	39.8	16.6	7.2	475
Sufficient rest	30.8	46.5	19.1	3.4	474
Daily teeth brushing	67.4	14.9	9.1	8.5	468
Sufficient fresh air	52.7	37.7	8.2	1.3	474
Protection from cold	54.4	32.4	10.1	3.0	472
Not overworking	21.3	30.3	30.5	17.9	475
Not overeating	23.9	34.8	22.4	18.8	473

* Refers to wearing a seat-belt while travelling in the front seat of a car. This was required by law at the time of interview.
Source: McCluskey, D. (1989).

From their responses to the second list of behaviours, it was found (table 14.2) that a majority of the respondents – in most instances a large majority – practised the specified health behaviours always or most of the time. It must be conceded, however, that for many people these practices may not have been the result of conscious decisions to promote their health. With the exception of seat-belt use, the actions may have been taken in the interest of personal appearance or again, they may have been habits acquired in childhood. In short, for many these practices may have represented *latent* health behaviours.

It was found that of the health behaviours, annual medical and dental check-ups were less commonly rated as important to health than such measures as getting enough fresh air, having sufficient rest, taking physical exercise, not eating too much, not being overweight and not overworking. Further, it emerged that the more importance attached to a particular health behaviour, the more frequently it tended to be practised.

As many as two thirds reported that they engaged in some form of physical activity outside work. The activities most frequently mentioned were walking and participation in games. Among other activities referred to were swimming, gardening, cycling and jogging. An interesting though not unexpected finding was that as the amount of physical exercise involved in their occupations decreased, the more frequently the respondents tended to engage in physical activities outside work. For example, of those who stated that their occupations involved a lot of physical work or exercise, 50 per cent reported that they engaged in physical activities outside of work; the same was true of 85 per cent of those who said their occupations entailed no physical work or exercise.

Particular attention was given to patterns of cigarette smoking. For many years there has been a steady decline in the prevalence of cigarette smoking in Ireland. In two national samples, one surveyed in 1998 and a second in 2002, the proportion of regular or occasional cigarette smokers in the adult population dropped from 31 per cent (1998) to 27 per cent (2002) (Friel et al., 1999; Centre for Health Promotion Studies, 2003). In the present study, 185 respondents (39 per cent) reported being regular smokers. Only 12 per cent of these claimed to have made a persistent attempt to give up the habit – this was usually for health reasons.

Non-smokers were much more likely than smokers to perceive cigarette smoking as a serious threat to a smoker's health and this was particularly true for former smokers (table 14.3). Non-smokers, too, were more likely to see cigarette *smoke* (passive smoking) as a serious threat to a non-smoker's health.

Socio-psychological influences
The Health Belief Model suggests that people who perceive themselves as susceptible to disease are more likely than others to take preventive action. Two rough measures of perceived susceptibility were employed in the study. The

Table 14.3 **Perceived threat of cigarette smoking to a smoker's health by cigarette smoking practices**

Cigarette Smoking Practice	Very serious threat	Serious threat	Fairly serious threat	Slight threat	No threat	N = 474
A regular smoker	25.4	22.2	33.0	10.8	8.6	185
Never a regular smoker	53.5	24.0	12.0	6.0	4.5	200
Non-smoker – formerly a regular smoker	59.6	22.5	10.0	4.5	3.4	89

Source: McCluskey (1989).

respondents were asked (i) to what extent they worried about becoming ill compared with most of their acquaintances, and (ii) what were the chances of their having to spend at least four days in bed because of illness during the succeeding twelve months. Their assessments were taken as rough measures of their perceived personal susceptibility to illness in general. It might be expected, therefore, that the more worried respondents were about becoming ill and the greater their perceived likelihood of having to spend a minimum of four days in bed, then the greater the probability that they would engage in some form of health behaviour. In neither case was such a relationship found.

A unidimensional Health Locus of Control (HLC) scale was employed as a measure of the respondents' beliefs that their health is determined by their own behaviour or by factors over which they have no control such as luck or chance. Based on the extent of their agreement/disagreement with six statements, such as, 'If I take care of myself I can avoid illness', the respondents were allocated to five categories ranging from high internals (those feeling most in control) to high externals (the most fatalistic). No consistent pattern was found between the respondents' HLC scores and whether they did or did not engage in health behaviour. However, it did emerge that those who were most fatalistic in their attitudes to health and illness (high externals) were the least likely to take any form of preventive action.

Illness behaviour
Illness behaviour denotes those actions which people take when they feel ill. Typically, these include complaining and requesting advice from members of their social networks, relatives or friends, and seeking consultation with health professionals.

David Tuckett (1976) has observed that many people with symptoms, often serious symptoms, do not seek medical help. He cites studies in both Britain and the United States where it was found that roughly for every person in care with a given condition, there was at least one, and in many cases several other persons outside care, with a symptom that was regarded as equally serious by the doctors who carried out the studies. Such evidence has drawn attention to the existence of what has been termed a *clinical* or *symptom iceberg* (Last, 1963; Hannay, 1979). Levels of ill health regularly treated among the population represent just the tip of an iceberg with a much larger proportion submerged or hidden. Thus, as Tuckett (1976) has demonstrated, whether studies are done in a free service as in the British National Health Service, or in a fee for service as in the United States, there is always a very large number of individuals with serious health problems who have not sought medical help.

Blaxter (1990) notes that in surveys most participants report themselves as being in good health. This was true of the respondents in the present study: 52 per cent reported that in general in the past their health had always been good and a further 39 per cent that it had been good most of the time. These findings are broadly similar to those of recent large-scale studies in Ireland (Friel et al., 1999; Centre for Health Promotion Studies, 2003). Again, when asked about their health status in the two weeks prior to interview, 37 per cent rated it as having been excellent and 47 per cent rated it as having been good. A minority (15 per cent) assessed their health as having been less than good during the same period.

Blaxter (1990) argues that defining oneself as being in good health does not necessarily exclude the presence of disease or symptoms. She records that in her own study many disabled and/or elderly people insisted on calling their health excellent even though this seemed an optimistic definition. Obviously, she comments, what these people were saying was 'my health is excellent considering my advanced years' or 'despite my disability'. The findings of the present study lend some support to this argument: though, in general, younger respondents were more likely than older respondents to define their health as favourable, differences were not pronounced.

If number of days confined to bed due to illness is taken as a measure of ill-health then most of the respondents in the study would appear to have enjoyed good health in the recent past. Only one third stated that they had spent at least one day in bed because of illness in the twelve months prior to interview and most of these had been confined to bed for less than a week. Indeed only 12 per cent of all respondents had spent a week or more in bed because of illness during the previous year.

To discover the respondents' most recent illness experiences they were first of all asked in open-ended questions what disease conditions they had experienced in the two weeks before interview. Then, to help jog their memories, they were presented with a checklist of 15 common symptoms and requested to indicate which, if any, they had experienced during the same period. Bringing together the information derived from both questions it emerged that over half (53 per cent) had experienced at least one illness or symptom in the two weeks prior to interview. The most frequently reported symptoms were headache (23 per cent), backache (14 per cent), sleeplessness (12 per cent), indigestion (12 per cent), stomach upset (12 per cent), and cough (11 per cent).

Though the above findings might suggest that illness, defined as the presence of symptoms, may have been a fairly frequent occurrence for very many in the sample population, at the same time it must be remembered that a very large minority (47 per cent) reported having experienced no symptoms in the specified two-week period. These results do not point therefore to illness experience being anything like as frequent a phenomenon as was found in a number of British and American studies (see Tuckett, 1976; Scambler, 1997a). This may be explained, to some extent, by the fact that the check-list of symptoms presented to the respondents was somewhat limited – a more extensive list might have called to memory a larger number of illness experiences. It may well be, of course, that differences in reporting symptomatic episodes are related to cultural definitions: what in one population is perceived as worthy of mention, may in another be considered too trivial to report. It is also conceivable that people in Ireland are somewhat reluctant to admit to illness experiences and in this respect resemble their Irish American cousins who Zola found tended to under-report symptoms, as described above.

Studies of illness behaviour indicate that the decision to consult a doctor in response to symptoms is a relatively rare occurrence for most people (Wadsworth, et al. 1971; Hannay, 1979). Jones (1994) cites evidence showing that a large and growing number of conditions are self-treated by lay people through the use of medicines from the chemist (pharmacist). The study being discussed here revealed similar patterns. Since most of the illnesses or symptoms were of a mild or non-serious nature, it is not surprising to find that only a small proportion (18 per cent) had consulted a doctor. Just over 39 per cent had taken patent medicines, and a further 18 per cent had simply stayed in bed or treated themselves with some form of home remedy. Almost 39 per cent had taken no action whatsoever. (Percentages sum to more than 100 since a number of respondents took more than one form of action.) The probability of having consulted a doctor was associated with age and the number of symptoms reported: respondents aged 35 years and over and respondents who had experienced three or more symptoms were more likely to have sought medical advice.

Dale Tussing of the Economic and Social Research Institute (ESRI), in a national survey in the Republic of Ireland (1985), found that two thirds of the sample population had consulted a GP at least once in 1980. In a later ESRI study, a somewhat smaller proportion of its sample (56 per cent) was found to have at least one GP consultation in 1987 (Nolan, 1991). In the present study it emerged that, for the 12 month period prior to interview, 61 per cent of the respondents for whom there was complete information had consulted a doctor, whether GP or other. The pattern of consultation was related to past experience of major illness: a significantly greater proportion of respondents who had sustained serious illness than of others reported that they had sought medical help, 77 per cent compared with 56 per cent.

The overwhelming majority of the respondents (87 per cent) reported that they had a regular doctor. Most, too, were in easy reach of the surgery: 54 per cent would usually arrive there in less than 15 minutes and a further 25 per cent from 15 to 29 minutes. However, 44 per cent stated they would have to wait at least half-an-hour before the consultation took place. Moreover, those who took longest to get to the surgery would usually have to wait longest for a consultation. A study in England (Kesl and Shepherd, 1965) has suggested that some persons rarely consult a doctor because they are too busy to do so and that people have to wait too long in doctors' surgeries. In the present study it was found that as reported waiting time increased, the proportion having an annual medical check-up decreased, though the differences were small. Nevertheless, it seems unlikely that in the absence of symptoms individuals will avail themselves of a medical check-up if it is perceived as making considerable demands on their time.

Two thirds (66 per cent) of the respondents indicated that, when ill, they would seek the opinion of another person as to whether or not they should consult a doctor. This significant other, who in almost all cases was a family member, usually a spouse, was commonly recognised as playing an important role in their decision making. This supports the claim of Freidson (1970) that the use of health services is very much influenced by what he calls a *lay referral system* – a network of close relatives and friends from whom advice will be sought in relation to illness.

One fifth (20 per cent) of the respondents had sought advice from a chemist (pharmacist) when ill. The illnesses were generally of a non-serious nature: colds and flu, sort throat, stomach trouble etc. It also emerged that 13 per cent had sought help from practitioners of alternative/complementary medicine: faith healers, herbalists, acupuncturists and persons with a religious cure. Most claimed that they had benefited considerably from contact with such sources.

Macro approach: age and gender

The principal findings of the study have been presented and variations in behaviour have been analysed from a micro perspective, that is, in terms of the personal characteristics of the respondents and of their health and illness experiences. A macro approach follows in which three of the socio-demographic variations in the respondents' health and illness behaviour are examined: age, gender and socio-economic status.

Health behaviour

It has been observed that participation in health behaviour is associated with both age and gender (Blaxter, 1990; Weiss and Lonnquist, 1999; Cockerham, 1998). A similar picture emerged from the study being discussed here (table 14.4). Older respondents, both male and female, appeared more concerned than younger respondents about their general health in that they were more inclined to have an annual medical check-up and to ensure that they had suffi- cient rest. On the other hand, dental care received considerably more attention from younger respondents: they were much more likely to report that they had a yearly dental examination and that they brushed their teeth at least once a day. However, this association between age and attention to dental health may be explained largely by older respondents being more likely to have had dentures fitted; the *Happy Heart National Survey* found than only half of those in its sample had most of their own teeth – the mean age of having dentures fitted was 31.6 years (Irish Heart Foundation, 1994).

Women would appear to have a healthier lifestyle than men. In general, they were more likely to have an annual medical check-up, to have a yearly dental examination and to brush their teeth every day. Concern with dental care was especially characteristic of young women. Significantly, women of all ages were much more likely to report that they were observing a diet to control their weight; the difference was striking for those under 35 years – 26 per cent of women compared with 4 per cent of men. Arguably, however, this may have as much to do with physical appearance as with health. Only in one respect did men appear to have a healthier lifestyle – at all age levels, they were more likely to indicate that they took sufficient exercise.

Smoking practices were found to vary with both age and gender. Regular cigarette smoking was highest for respondents under 35 years of age, it decreased somewhat for those aged 35 to 64 years and dropped considerably for those aged 65 and over. So, too, a greater proportion of men reported that they were regular cigarette smokers when interviewed.

Illness behaviour

Since health status tends to decline with age it was not surprising that older respondents were less disposed to assess their past health as having always been good and further, that they more frequently reported that they had experienced major illness and that they had consulted a doctor during the previous year and in the two weeks prior to interview. Younger respondents, in contrast, exhibited less anxiety about becoming ill and were less likely to consider themselves susceptible to illness.

Table 14.4 **Participation in specific health behaviours by gender and age**

Health behaviour	Frequency	Gender	Age (%)								
			18–24	25–34	35–44	45–54	55–64	65+	All Ages	N
Medical check-up	At least once a year	M	7.9	14.3	25.6	34.5	39.4	44.0	25.3	217
		F	17.5	22.2	29.4	31.8	45.9	40.0	30.4	257
Dental check-up	At least once a year	M	34.2	24.5	18.6	32.1	6.1	8.0	21.3	216
		F	62.5	40.7	35.3	23.3	13.5	—	29.0	255
Daily teeth brushing	Always	M	76.3	67.3	52.3	58.6	39.4	34.8	56.9	216
		F	92.5	90.7	78.8	75.0	66.7	50.0	76.2	252
Sufficient exercise	Always	M	44.7	44.9	50.0	41.4	39.4	40.0	44.0	218
		F	27.5	25.9	35.3	36.4	18.9	31.1	30.0	257
Sufficient rest	Always	M	23.7	18.4	20.5	24.1	36.4	66.7	28.6	217
		F	10.0	18.5	29.4	36.4	48.6	53.3	32.7	257
Protection from cold	Always	M	47.4	30.6	38.6	48.3	45.5	68.0	44.0	218
		F	51.3	59.3	69.7	53.5	59.6	84.4	63.4	254
Wearing a seat belt	Always	M	55.3	55.1	41.9	41.4	39.4	28.0	45.2	217
		F	50.0	42.6	50.0	52.3	45.9	42.2	47.1	257
Not over-eating	Always	M	21.6	18.4	18.2	20.7	21.9	20.0	20.8	216
		F	20.0	27.8	23.5	18.2	35.1	33.3	26.5	257
Dietary control of weight	—	M	5.3	2.1	21.4	17.2	27.3	12.5	13.6	214
		F	25.0	26.4	24.2	34.9	42.9	24.4	29.4	252

Source: McCluskey (1989).

Gender differences also emerged in personal health assessments and in illness behaviour. Men tended to rate their general health in the past more favourably; they also appeared less anxious about becoming ill and were more optimistic about their future health status. Women, on the other hand, were more likely to have consulted a doctor in the previous twelve months and to have sought medical help in the two weeks prior to interview.

Macro approach: socio-economic status

William Cockerham (1998), who uses the terms social class and socio-economic status interchangeably, has observed that socio-economic status is one of the strongest and most consistent predictors of a person's health and life expectancy, that lower socio-economic groups have the poorest health. Moreover, as has already been pointed out, people of lower socio-economic status are less likely to engage in behaviour commonly held as conducive to good health, for example they are more likely to smoke cigarettes but less likely to make use of preventive services.

Cockerham notes that socio-economic status typically consists of measures of income, occupational status and level of education. He adds that, while income and occupational status are important, the strongest single predictor of good health appears to be education. Well-educated people are generally the best informed about the merits of a healthy lifestyle and the advantages of seeking preventive care. Two measures of socio-economic status were employed in the present study: occupational status and level of educational attainment, that is, the number of years spent in full-time education. Married women and widows were classified in terms of the occupational status of their husbands and young people, not yet employed, in terms of the occupational status of their fathers.

Health behaviour
No significant relationship was found between the frequency of having an annual medical check-up and either occupational status or level of educational attainment. But, it did emerge that respondents from the professional and managerial classes were four times more likely than those from manual working-class backgrounds to report that they had an annual dental check-up. The likelihood of having an annual dental examination also increased as the level of educational attainment rose, as did the brushing of one's teeth every day. However, just as the relationship between age and attention to dental health may be largely explained by older respondents being more likely to have had dentures fitted, similarly the association between social class and a concern with dental care may be explained, to some extent at least, by the greater likelihood of those in upper socio-economic groups having most of their own teeth and no dentures, as was found in the *Happy Heart National Survey* (Irish Heart Foundation, 1994). It emerged also that respondents with higher levels of education were more likely to report that they always wore a seat-belt when travelling in the front seat of a car, and that they engaged in physical exercise in the interest of their health. So, too, the likelihood of taking physical exercise was greater for those in non-manual groups than for those from manual back-grounds. In contrast, significantly higher proportions of regular cigarette smokers were found among those in the manual working classes than in non-manual occupations and among those with lower levels of educational attainment. These findings, in respect of cigarette smoking, are consistent with those of the National Health and Lifestyle Surveys (Friel et al., 1999; Centre for Health Promotion Studies, 2003).

Illness behaviour

Significant class differences also emerged in the respondents' illness behaviour. Respondents from manual occupational backgrounds and respondents with lower educational levels were found to be higher utilisers of medical services, in that they were more likely to have sought a doctor's help for symptoms experienced in the two weeks prior to interview. In general, respondents of lower socio-economic status appeared less optimistic about their future health than those of higher status levels: they worried more about becoming ill and perceived themselves as more susceptible to illness. This behaviour and these attitudes of working-class respondents most likely reflect their greater health needs (see chapter 5 above).

Conclusion

Thomas McKeown (1979) maintains that the way forward to improve the health of populations in the developed world is through changes in individual's behaviour: 'Both health and quality of life are improved by taking exercise, avoiding tobacco and other drugs, and limiting consumption of alcohol and food. As these are now the main determinants of health it is hard to believe that society will not wish to create conditions under which such practices are encouraged' (McKeown, 1979: 183). However, as argued in chapter 5, behaviour cannot be separated from its social context – certain living and working conditions severely restrict an individual's ability to choose a healthy lifestyle. More important, an emphasis on behaviour may draw attention away from the structural and material factors which, more than any other, explain health inequalities. As a result, health promotion policy may be interpreted in the narrow sense of changing behaviour while ignoring the influence on health of the economic, social and ecological factors highlighted at the start of this chapter.

Ian Rees Jones (1999) has related that in recent years sociological critiques of health promotion have questioned its ideological foundation. According to Jones, critics argue that the glossing-over of the problem of structure and agency has led to the re-introduction of individualistic and 'victim blaming' tendencies and that health promotion workers might be the unwilling vehicles for new forms of social control within advanced liberalism. He refers to the work of Bunton et al. (1995) which categorises sociological critiques under three headings: socio-structural, surveillance and consumption based. To these, Rees Jones adds a fourth of his own: system-based critiques.

Socio-structural critiques propose that within health promotion the importance of social, political and physical environments in people's lives is neglected. Surveillance critiques imply that health promotion and public health workers are involved in population surveillance which, in effect, is an extension of the medical gaze from individuals to communities, as elaborated by Armstrong (1995). Consumption critiques, Rees Jones argues, lead to health promotion workers beginning to resemble the 'new cultural intermediaries', identified by Bourdieu (1984), promoting and privileging specific lifestyles. Rees Jones refers to a fourth critique of health promotion developed by Scambler and Scambler (1995), which argues that health promotion work is mainly limited to securing change at the level of operational work, leaving factors at political and structural level unaddressed.

Margaret Blaxter (2003) maintains that the biological is an awkward topic in inequality studies. Ever since the publication of the Black Report (Department of Health and Social Security (UK), 1980) research on class inequality, faced with the biological, has defensively been intent on emphasising the materialist view. One reason, she suggests, for the unease about the biological in inequalities research is that the biological can be seen as too redolent of the medical model. Even though the medical model may be something of a sociological caricature, she argues that teaching that it is the antithesis of the social model of health has tended to remove the physicality of the body.

Blaxter suggests the metaphor of *health capital* may help in our understanding of the interplay between biological and social factors in the patterning of health and illness. As Blaxter (2003: 79–80) expresses it: 'A genetic stock of health capital is laid down at conception: in utero, at birth and in early infancy it is elaborated and the basis is provided for health in later life. Opportunities exist throughout life for the augmentation or depletion of this capital, through education, family life and occupation.' Blaxter goes on to elaborate on the many ways this capital may be depleted – by smoking, by unwise eating, by work dangers and stresses, by environmental damage, by accidental infection and trauma. She also points out that it can be augmented by 'healthy' behaviour or the deliberate search for 'fitness' or by positive, life-enhancing circumstances.

To the author, Blaxter's notion of health capital would appear to provide a very useful tool in future analyses of the phenomena of health and illness behaviour.

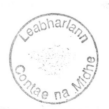

References

Abel-Smith, B. (1960) *A History of the Nursing Profession*. London: Heinemann.

Advisory Group on the Risk Equalisation Scheme (1998) *Report of the Advisory Group on the Risk Equalisation Scheme*. Dublin: Stationery Office..

Aiken, L. H., S. P. Clarke, R. B. Cheung, D. M. Sloane and J. H. Silber (2003) 'Educational levels of hospital nurses and surgical patient mortality', *Journal of the American Medical Association* 290 (12): 1617–23.

AIM (Association Internationale de la Mutualité) (1994) *AIM's Mission*. Geneva: AIM.

Amárach Consulting (2003) *The Private Health Insurance Market in Ireland*. Dublin: Health Insurance Authority.

An Bórd Altranais (1991) *Nurse Education and Training Consultative Document*. Dublin: An Bórd Altranais.

An Bórd Altranais (1994) *The Future of Nurse Education and Training in Ireland*. Dublin: An Bórd Altranais.

An Bórd Altranais (1997) *Continuing Professional Education for Nurses: A Framework*. Dublin: An Bórd Altranais.

An Bórd Altranais (1999) *Review of the Scope of Practice for Nursing and Midwifery: Interim Report*. Dublin: An Bórd Altranais.

Annandale, E. (1998) *The Sociology of Health and Medicine*. Cambridge: Polity.

Anon. (1955) *The Irish Nurses Magazine* 23 (2): 8.

Armstrong, D. (1994) *Outline of Sociology as Applied to Medicine*. Oxford: Butterworth-Heinemann.

Armstrong, D. (1995) 'The rise of surveillance medicine', *Sociology of Health and Illness* 7 (3): 393–404.

Balanda, K. and J. Wilde (2001) *Inequalities in Mortality: A Report on All-Ireland Mortality Data*. Dublin: Institute of Public Health in Ireland.

Barrington, R. (1987) *Health, Medicine and Politics in Ireland 1900–1970*. Dublin: IPA.

Barry, J. (1989) *The Travellers' Health Status Study: Vital Statistics of the Travelling People 1987*. Dublin: Health Research Board.

Barry, J., H. Sinclair, A. Kelly, R. O'Loughlin, D. Handy and J. O'Dowd (2001) *Inequalities in Health in Ireland: Hard Facts*. Dublin: Health Research Board.

Bassett, C. (1992) 'The integration of research in the clinical setting: obstacles and solutions. A review of the literature', *Nursing Practice* 6 (1): 4–8.

Bayley, M. (1973) *Mental Handicap and Community Care*. London: Routledge & Kegan Paul.

Becker, H. S. et al. (1961), *Boys in White*. Chicago: University of Chicago Press.

Becker, M. (1979) 'Psychosocial aspects of health-related behaviour', pp. 253–74 in H. Freeman, S. Levine and L. Reeder (eds), *Handbook of Medical Sociology*. Englewood Cliffs: Prentice-Hall.

Becker, M. and L. Maiman (1983) 'Models of health-related behaviour', pp. 539–68 in D. Mechanic (ed.), *Handbook of Health, Health Care and the Health Professions*. New York: Free Press.

Bensman, J. and I. Gerver, (1963) 'Crime and punishment in the factory: the function of deviancy in maintaining a social system', *American Sociological Review* 38 (4): 448–89.

Berk, M. L. and A. C. Monheit (1992) 'The concentration of health expenditures: an update', *Health Affairs* 11: 145–9.

Biggart, J. H. (1968) 'The challenge of nurse education', *International Nursing Review* 15 (4), 292–307.

Blackwell, J., E. O'Shea, G. Moane and P. Murray (1992) *Care Provision and Cost Measurement*. Dublin: ESRI.

Blane, D. (1997) 'Inequality and social class', pp. 103–20 in G. Scambler (ed.), *Sociology as Applied to Medicine*. London: W. B. Saunders.

Blanshard, P. (1954) *The Irish and Catholic Power: An American Interpretation*. London: Derek Verschoyle.

Blau, P. (1963) *The Dynamics of Bureaucracy*. Chicago: University of Chicago Press.

Blaxter, M. (1984) 'Equity and consultation rates in general practice', *British Medical Journal* 288: 1963–7.

Blaxter, M. (1990) *Health and Lifestyles*. London: Tavistock/Routledge.

Blaxter, M. (2003) 'Biology, social class and inequalities in health: their synthesis in "health capital"', pp. 69–83 in S. Williams, L. Birke and G. Bendelow (eds), *Debating Biology*. London: Routledge.

Bonda, J. and S. Bonda (1986) *Sociology and Health Care*. Edinburgh: Churchill Livingstone.

Bourdieu, P. (1984) *Distinction: A Social Critique of the Judgement of Taste*. London: Routledge.

Bowling, A. (1997) *Research Methods in Health. Buckingham*: Open University Press.

Brearley, P., J. Gibbons, A. Miles, E. Topliss and G. Woods (1978) *The Social Context of Health Care*. Oxford: Martin Robertson.

Browne, N. (1986) *Against the Tide*. Dublin: Gill & Macmillan.

Bucher, R. and A. Strauss (1961) 'Professions in process', *American Journal of Sociology* 66: 32–4.

Buckley, A. D. (1987) '"On the club": friendly societies in Ireland', *Irish Economic and Social History* 14: 39–58.

Bunton, R., S. Nettleton and R. Burrows (1995) *The Sociology of Health Promotion*. London: Routledge.

BUPA Ireland (1996) *Essential Scheme Rules and Table of Benefits*. n.d. (November 1996).

Burke, S., C. Keenaghan, D. O'Donovan and B. Quirke (2004) *Health in Ireland: An Unequal State.* Dublin: Public Health Alliance.

Byrne, P. S. and B. E. Long (1976) *Doctors Talking to Patients.* London: HMSO.

Callan J. and B. Farrell (1991) *Women's Participation in the Labour Market.* Dublin: NESC.

Cassell, E. (1986) 'The changing concept of the ideal physician', *Daedalus* 115: 196.

Central Statistics Office (2004) Census 2002 http://www.cso.ie/

Centre for Health Promotion Studies (2003) *The National Health and Lifestyles Surveys.* Dublin: Health Promotion Unit, Department of Health and Children.

Chandler, A. D. (1962) *Strategy and Structure: Chapters in the History of the Industrial Enterprise.* Cambridge, MA: MIT Press.

Chavasse, J. (1998) 'Policy as an influence on public health nursing education in the Republic of Ireland', *Journal of Advanced Nursing* 28: 172–7.

Cherichovsky, D. (1995). 'Health system reforms in industrialized democracies: an emerging paradigm', *Milbank Quarterly* 73: 339–72.

Chubb, B. (1992) *The Government and Politics of Ireland,* 3rd edn. Harlow: Longman.

Chun an Aire Sláinte (1996). 'To the Minister of Health', 17 December (typescript).

Clamp, C. G. L. (1994) *Resources for Nursing Research.* London: Library Association.

Clarke, D. J. (1996) 'Where to from here?: The emerging issues', Association of Nurse Teachers' Conference, September, 1996. Dublin: Association of Nurse Teachers.

Clarke, E. (1990) 'Setting up our own group home', *Frontline* 7: 11–12.

Cleary, A. and M. P. Treacy (eds) (1997) *The Sociology of Health and Illness in Ireland.* Dublin: University College Dublin Press.

Cockerham, W. (1995) *Medical Sociology,* 6th edn. Englewood Cliffs NJ: Prentice-Hall.

Cockerham, W. (1998) *Medical Sociology,* 7th edn. New Jersey: Prentice-Hall.

Colgan, A. (1997) 'People with disabilities and the health services', pp. 111–25 in J. Robins (ed.) *Reflections on Health.* Dublin: Department of Health.

Commission on Financial Management and Control Systems in the Health Service (2003) *Report* (Brennan Report). Dublin: Stationery Office.

Commission on Health Funding (1989) *Report.* Dublin: Stationery Office.

Commission on the Status of People with Disabilities (1996) *A Strategy for Equality.* Dublin: Stationery Office.

Condell, S. (1998) *Changes in the Professional Role of Nurses in Ireland: 1980–1997: A Report Prepared for the Commission on Nursing.* Dublin: Stationery Office.

Connolly, C. et al. (1998) 'Attitudes of young men and women to breastfeeding', *Irish Medical Journal* 91 (3): 88–9.

Consultative Council on the General Hospital Services (1968) *Outline of the Future Hospital System: Report* (*Fitzgerald Report*). Dublin: Stationery Office.

Cooper, M and S. Smyth (1997). 'Relationships between VHI and civil servants far from healthy', *Sunday Times* (Irish edn) 5 January: 6.

Council of the European Communities (1977) 'Council Directive of 27 June 1977 concerning the mutual recognition of diplomas, certificates and other evidence of formal qualifications of nurses responsible for general care, including measures to facilitate the effective exercise of this right of establishment and freedom to provide services (77/452/EEC)', *Official Journal of the European Communities* 20 (No L 176, 1977): 1–13.

Council of the European Communities (1989) 'Council Directive of 10 October 1989, (89/595/EEC) amending Directives concerning the mutual recognition of diplomas, certificates and other evidence of formal qualifications of nurses responsible for general care, including measures to facilitate the effective exercise of this right of establishment and freedom to provide services, and amending Directive 77/453/EEC concerning the co-ordination of provisions laid down by law, regulation or administrative action in respect of the activities of nurses responsible for general care', *Official Journal of the European Communities*, No. L 341/30, article 2, para. 4.

Cousins, M. (1995) *Policy Analysis of Submissions*, prepared for the Commission on the Status of People with Disabilities.

Cowley, S., A. Bergen, K. Young and A. Kavanagh (1995) 'Exploring needs assessment in community nursing', *Health Visitor* 68 (8): 319–21.

Cullen, G. (2002) *Perinatal Statistics for 1999*. Dublin: ESRI, HIPE and NPRS Unit.

Currie, Austin (1996) 'Speech by Austin Currie, TD, Minister of State at Department of Health, on Adjournment, Wednesday, 20 November 1996.' (typescript).

Curry, John (1993) *Irish Social Services*. Dublin: IPA.

Daly, A. and D. Walsh (2001) *Activities of the Irish Psychiatric Services 2000*. Dublin: Health Research Board.

Daly, A. and D. Walsh (2002) *Irish Psychiatric Hospitals and Units Census 2001*. Dublin: Health Research Board.

Daly, M. E. (1999) 'An atmosphere of sturdy independence: The state and the Dublin hospitals in the 1930s', pp. 234–52 in E. Malcolm and G. Jones (eds), *Medicine, Disease and the State in Ireland 1650–1940*. Cork: Cork University Press.

Daniels, Norman (1985) *Just Health Care*. Cambridge, UK: Cambridge University Press.

Daniels, Norman (1988) *Am I My Parent's Keeper?* New York: Oxford University Press.

Daniels, Norman, Donald Light and Ron Caplan (1996). *Benchmarks of Fairness in Health Care Reform*. New York: Oxford University Press.

Davey Smith, G., M. Bartley and D. Blane (1990) 'The Black Report on socio-economic inequalities in health 10 years on', *British Medical Journal* 301: 373–7.

Davis, F. (1972) *Illness Interaction and the Self*. Belmont CA: Wadsworth.

Deeny, J. (1949) *The Irish Nurses Magazine* 16 (11): 2–5.

Deeny, J. (1989) *To Cure and To Care: Memoirs of a Chief Medical Officer*. Dublin: Glendale Press.

Deloitte & Touche (2001) *Value for Money Audit of the Irish Health System*. Dublin: Deloitte and Touche.

Denton, J. (1978) Medical Sociology. Boston: Houghton Mifflin.

Department of Education and Science (1998) Press Release: 'Major initiative in special education services.' Dublin: Department of Education and Science.

Department of Education and Science (2001) *Report of the Task Force on Autism.* Dublin: Department of Education and Science.

Department of Health (1965) *Report of the Commission of Enquiry on Mental Handicap.* Dublin: Stationery Office.

Department of Health (1966a) *The Health Services and Their Further Development* (White Paper). Dublin: Stationery Office.

Department of Health (1966b) *Commission of Enquiry on Mental Illness.* Dublin: Stationery Office.

Department of Health (1974) *Training and Employing the Handicapped.* Dublin: Department of Health.

Department of Health (1980) *Working Party on General Nursing.* Dublin: Stationery Office.

Department of Health (1984) *The Psychiatric Services: Planning for the Future.* Dublin: Stationery Office.

Department of Health (1985–91) *Perinatal Statistics Reports* (annual) Dublin: Stationery Office.

Department of Health (1986) *Health: The Wider Dimensions.* Dublin: Department of Health.

Department of Health (1992) *Green Paper on Mental Health.* Dublin: Stationery Office.

Department of Health (1994a) *Shaping a Healthier Future: A Strategy for Effective Healthcare in the 1990s.* Dublin: Stationery Office.

Department of Health (1994b) *White Paper on Mental Health.* Dublin: Stationery Office.

Department of Health (1996) 'BUPA products', press release, 20 Dec.

Department of Health (1997a) *Services to Persons with a Mental Handicap /Intellectual Disability: An Assessment of Need, 1997–2001.* Dublin: Stationery Office..

Department of Health (1997b) *Enhancing the Partnership: Report of the Working Group on implementation of the Health Strategy in relation to Persons with a Mental Handicap.* Dublin: Stationery Office.

Department of Health (1997c) 'Noonan announces agreement with BUPA Ireland', press release, 17 January.

Department of Health and Children (1998) *White Paper: Private Health Insurance.* Dublin: Stationery Office.

Department of Health and Children (2001a) *Quality and Fairness: A Health System for You.* Dublin: Stationery Office.

Department of Health and Children (2001b) *Primary Care: A New Direction.* Dublin: Stationery Office.

Department of Health and Children (2001c) *Your Views About Health: Report on Consultation.* Dublin: Stationery Office.

Department of Health and Children (2002) *Acute Hospital Bed Capacity: A National Review*. Dublin: Stationery Office.

Department of Health and Children (2003a) *Health Statistics 2002*. Dublin: Stationery Office.

Department of Health and Children (2003b) *Report of the National Task Force on Medical Staffing* (Hanly Report). Dublin: Department of Health and Children.

Department of Health and Children (2003c) *The Health Service Reform Programme*. Dublin: Stationery Office.

Department of Health and Social Security (UK) (1980) *Inequalities in Health: Report of a Research Working Group* (The Black Report). London: HMSO.

Department of Justice, Equality and Law Reform (1998) Employment Equality Act.

Department of Justice, Equality and Law Reform (2000) Equal Status Act.

Department of Justice, Equality and Law Reform (2001) Disability Bill.

Department of Local Government and Public Health (1936), *The Hospitals Commission, First General Report*. Dublin: Stationery Office.

Department of the Environment (1991) *Building Regulations. Technical Guidance Document M: Access for Disabled People*. Dublin: Stationery Office..

Digby, A. and N. Bosanquet (1988) 'Doctors and patients in an era of national health insurance and private practice, 1913–1938', *Economic History Review* 41: 74–94.

Director of the Office of Equality Investigations Cases. www. odei.ie

Ditton, J. (1977) 'Learning to fiddle the customers – an essay on the organised production of part-time theft', *Sociology of Work & Occupations* 4 (4): 427–50.

Dobbin, Frank (1994) *Forging Industrial Policy: the United States, Britain, and France in the Railway Age*. New York: Cambridge University Press.

Douglas, Mary (1966) *Purity and Danger*. London: Routledge & Kegan Paul.

Elias, Norbert (1994) *The Civilising Process*, one-volume edn. Oxford: Blackwell.

Elms, R. R., B. Tierney and P. A. Boylan (1974) 'Irish nursing at the crossroads', *International Journal of Nursing Studies* 11: 163–72.

Elston M. and L. Doyal (1983) *The Changing Experience of Women: Health and Medicine* (unit 14). Milton Keynes: Open University Press.

Engel, G. (1977) 'The need for a new medical model: a challenge for biomedicine', *Science* 196: 129–36.

Enthoven, Alain (1988) *Theory and Practice of Managed Competition in Health Care Finance*. Amsterdam: North-Holland.

Epsom, J. (1978) 'The mobile health clinic: A report on the first year's work', pp. 107–13 in D. Tuckett and J. Kaufert (eds), *Basic Readings in Medical Sociology*. London: Tavistock.

European Commission (1996) *Communication of the Commission on Equality of Opportunity for People with Disabilities: A New European Disability Strategy*, COM (96). Brussels: European Commission.

Fahey, J. and P. Murray (1994) *Health and Autonomy among the Over-65s in Ireland*. Dublin: National Council For The Elderly.

Faughnan, P. (1997) 'A healthy voluntary sector: rhetoric or reality?', pp. 232–49 in J. Robins, (ed.) *Reflections on Health*. Dublin: Department of Health.

Faughnan, P. and S. O'Connor, (1980) *Major Issues in Planning Services for Mentally and Physically Handicapped Persons* (NESC Report No. 50). Dublin: Stationery Office.

Fealy, G. M. (2002a) 'A history of the provision and reform of general nurse education and training in Ireland, 1879–1994', PhD thesis, University College Dublin.

Fealy, G. M. (2002b) 'Aspects of curriculum policy in pre-registration nursing education in the Republic of Ireland: issues and reflections', *Journal of Advanced Nursing* 37 (6): 558–65.

Fildes, V. (1986) *Breasts, Bottles and Babies: A History of Infant Feeding*. Edinburgh: Edinburgh University Press.

Finch, J. (1990) 'The politics of community care in Britain', pp. 34–58 in C. Ungerson (ed.), *Gender and Caring: Work and Welfare in Britain and Scandinavia*. London: Wheatsheaf.

FitzGerald, Garret (1996) 'Proposed BUPA scheme is fatal for our health service', *The Irish Times*, 28 December.

Foucault, M. (1979) *Discipline and Punish: The Birth of the Prison*. New York: Vintage.

Foucault, M. (1980) *Power/Knowledge: Selected Interviews and Other Writings 1972–1977*. Brighton: Harvester.

Foyster, L. (1995) 'Supporting mothers: an inter-disciplinary approach', *Health Visitor* 68 (4): 151–2.

Freidson, E. (1970) *Professions of Medicine: A Study of The Sociology of Applied Knowledge*. New York: Dodd, Mead.

Friel, S., S. Nic Gabhainn and C. Kelleher (1999) *The National Health and Lifestyles Surveys*. Dublin: Department of Health and Children; Galway: National University of Ireland, Galway.

General Medical Service (Payments) Board (2004) *Report for the year ended 31 December 2003*.

General Nursing Council for Ireland (1923) *Regulations Made by the General Nursing Council*, Minutes of General Nursing Council for Ireland, 19 July.

General Nursing Council for Ireland (1926) Minutes of General Nursing Council for Ireland, 25 February 1920.

Gillespie, R. and R. Prior (1995) 'Health inequalities', pp. 195–212 in G. Moon and R. Gillespie (eds), *Society and Health*. London: Routledge.

Goldthorpe, J. (1992) 'The theory of industrialism and the Irish case', pp. 411–31 in J. Goldthorpe and C. Whelan (eds), *The Development of Industrial Society in Ireland*. Oxford: Oxford University Press.

Government of Ireland (1996) Statutory Instruments 1996. Nos 80–4. *Health Insurance Act, 1994. Regulations, 1996*. Dublin: Stationery Office.

Government of Ireland (1998) *A Blueprint for the Future: Report of the Commission on Nursing*. Dublin: Stationery Office.

Green, P. E. and D. S. Tull (1978) *Research for Marketing Decisions*. New Jersey: Prentice Hall.

Griffon, D. P. (1994) '"Crowning the edifice": Ethel Fenwick and state registration', *Nursing History Review.* 201–12.

Guidon, G. (1990) *Needs and Abilities: A policy for the intellectually disabled.* Dublin: Stationery Office.

Gustavsson, N. S. and E. A. Segal (1994) *Critical Issues in Child Welfare.* California: Sage.

Hanlon, Noel (1996) Letter to the Minister for Health, 20 November: 1–2.

Hannay, D. (1979) *The Symptom Iceberg: A Study of Community Health.* London: Routledge & Kegan Paul.

Harris, D. and S. Guten (1979) 'Health protective behaviour: An exploratory study', *Journal of Health and Social Behaviour* 20: 17–29.

Hart, N. (1985) 'The sociology of health and medicine', pp. 519–654 in M. Haralambos (ed.), *Sociology: New Directions.* Ormskirk, Lancs: Causeway.

Hasler, F. (1993) 'The place of information provision in the disability movement', in *Papers Presented at the National Disability Information Projects Conference.* London: Policy Studies Institute.

Hay, C. (1996) *Re-Stating Social and Political Change.* Buckingham: Open University Press.

Health Education Bureau (1987) *Promoting Health Through Public Policy.* Dublin: Health Education Bureau.

Health Research Board (1996) *National Intellectual Disability Database.* Dublin: Health Research Board.

Health Research Board (1988/1999) National Intellectual Disability Database. Dublin: HRB.

Health Research Board (2000) National Intellectual Disability Database. Dublin: HRB.

Hendriks, A. (1995) 'The concepts of non-discrimination and reasonable accommodation', in *Invisible Citizens.* Brussels: Secretariat of Disabled Persons.

Hensey, B. (1988) *The Health Services of Ireland*, 4th edn. Dublin: IPA.

Hildegarde, S. (1968) 'Professional socialisation in two baccalaureate programs', *Nursing Research* 17 (Sept./Oct.).

Horgan, J. (2000) *Noel Browne: Passionate Outsider.* Dublin: Gill & Macmillan.

House of Commons (1854) *Report of the Select Committee on Dublin Hospitals, Minutes of Evidence, Appendix and Index*, H.C. (383) xii.1.

House of Commons (1905) *Select Committee on the Registration of Nurses, together with the Proceedings of the Committee, Minutes of Evidence, Appendix and Index*, H.C. (281) vi.701 and 263.

Hsiao, William C. (1994) 'Marketization – the illusory magic pill', *Health Economics* 3: 351–7.

Hughes, Everett Charrington (1936) 'The ecological aspect of institutions', *American Sociological Review* 1: 180–92.

Hurley, M (1994) *A National Breastfeeding Policy for Ireland: A Report to the Minister for Health*. Dublin: Department of Health.

Hyde A. and M. Treacy (1999) 'Nurse education in the Republic of Ireland: negotiating a new educational space', pp. 89–108 in B. Connolly and A. Ryan (eds), *Women and Education in Ireland*, vol 1. Maynooth: Maynooth Adult Community Education.

Inglis, Tom (1987) *Moral Monopoly: The Catholic Church in Irish Society*. Dublin: Gill & Macmillan. (rev. edn, *Moral Monopoly: The Rise and Fall of the Catholic Church in Ireland*. Dublin: University College Dublin Press, 1998.)

Institute of Community Health Nursing (1994a) *Submission to the Department of Health on the Role of the Public Health Nurse*. Dublin: Institute of Community Health Nursing.

Institute of Community Health Nursing (1994b) *Submission on the Strategy Document: Shaping a Healthier Future*. Dublin: Institute of Community Health Nursing.

Irish Court Reports (1997) *O'Donoghue v the Minister for Health*, High Court.

Irish Court Reports (2001) *Sinnott v Minister for Education & Science*, Supreme Court.

Irish Heart Foundation (1994) *Happy Heart National Survey*. Dublin: Irish Heart Foundation.

Irish Patients' Association and Lansdowne Market Research (1999), *Omnibus Survey*.

Jones, L. (1994) *The Social Context of Health and Health Work*. Basingstoke: Macmillan.

Kalberg, Stephen (1980) 'Max Weber's types of rationality: Cornerstones for the analysis of rationalization process in history', *American Journal of Sociology* 97: 496–523.

Kasl, S. and S. Cobb (1966) 'Health behaviour, illness behaviour, and sick role behaviour', *Archives of Environmental Health* 12: 246–66.

Kelly, A. (1995) 'A public health nursing perspective', in H. Ferguson and P. Kenny (eds), *On Behalf of the Child*. Dublin: A. & A. Farmar.

Kelly, M. and B. Charlton (1995) 'The modern and postmodern in health promotion', in R. Bunton, S. Nettleton and R. Burrows (eds), *The Sociology of Health Promotion*. London: Routledge.

Kerr, C., J. Dunlop, F. Harbison and C. Myers (1973) *Industrialism and Industrial Man*. Harmondsworth: Penguin.

Kesl, N. and M. Shepherd (1965) 'the health and attitudes of people who seldom consult a doctor', *Medical Care* 3: 6–10.

Kinsella, S. (1997) 'Menni enterprises: do we belong?', *Frontline* 31: 8–9.

Kirkham, M. J. (1983) 'Labouring in the dark: limitations on the giving of information to enable patients to orientate themselves to the likely events and timescale of labour', pp. 81–100 in J. Wilson-Barnet (ed.), *Nursing Research: Ten Studies in Patient Care*. Chichester: Wiley.

Kramer, M. (1974) *Reality Shock: Why Nurses Leave Nursing*. Saint Louis, MO: C.V. Mosley.

Kramer, M., and C. Schmalenberg (1979) 'Bicultural training: a cost effective program', *Journal of Nursing Administration* Dec: 10–16.

Laffoy, M. (1997) 'Childhood accidents at home', *Irish Medical Journal* 90: 26–7.

Lally, C. (2002) 'Close Beaumont and start from scratch' (Interview with Dr David Hickey) *The Irish Times*, 19 Nov. 2002.

Lamont, Michele (1992) *Money, Morals and Manners: The Culture of the French and American Upper-Middle Class*. Chicago: University of Chicago Press.

Last, J. (1963) 'The clinical iceberg: completing the clinical picture in general practice', *Lancet* 2: 28–30.

Leahy, A., and M. Wiley (1998) (eds), *The Irish Health System in the 21 st Century*. Dublin: Oak Tree.

Leeuwenhorst Working Party (1974) 'The general practitioner in europe', *Journal of Royal College of General Practitioners* 27: 117.

Levenstein, J. H., J. B. Brown and W. W. Weston (1989) 'Patient-centred clinical interviewing', in M. Stewart and D. Roter (eds), *Communicating with Medical Patients*. New York: Sage.

Light, Donald W. (1992) 'The practice and ethics of risk-rated health insurance', *Journal of the American Medical Association* 271: 2503–8.

Light, Donald W. (1994) 'Comparative models of "health care" systems', pp. 455–69 in C. Conrad and R. Kern (eds), *The Sociology of Health and Illness: Critical Perspectives*. New York: St Martin's Press.

Light, Donald W. (1995) 'Homo economicus: escaping the traps of managed competition', *European Journal of Public Health* 5: 145–54.

Light, Donald W. (1996) 'An unhealthy tale of immorality', *Sunday Business Post*, 8 Dec.: 17.

Light, Donald W. (1997a) 'BUPA plans to threaten the social basis of health insurance', *The Irish Times*, 9 Jan.: 5.

Light, Donald W. (1997b) 'From managed competition to managed cooperation: theory and lessons from the British experience', *Millbank Quarterly* 75: 297–341.

Light, Donald W. (1999) 'The sociological character of markets in health care', pp. 394–408 in Gary L. Albrecht, Ray Fitzpatrick and Susan C. Scrimshaw (eds), *Handbook of Social Studies in Health and Medicine*. San Francisco: Sage.

Lynch, K. and E. McLaughlin (1995) 'Caring labour and love labour', pp. 250–94 in P. Clancy et al. (eds), *Sociological Perspectives*. Dublin: IPA.

MacCurtain, M. and M. O'Dowd (eds) (1991) *Women in Early Modern Ireland*. Edinburgh: Edinburgh University Press.

Macintosh, William Alex (1996) *Sociologies of Food and Nutrition*. New York and London: Plenum.

Macintyre, S. (1997) 'The Black Report and beyond: what are the issues?', *Social Science and Medicine* 44: 723–45.

Mackay, L. (1995) 'The nurse's role in giving nutritional advice', *Professional Nurse* 68 (7): 427–8.

Madden, P. J. (1994) 'The future education and training of nurses', *The New World of Irish Nursing* 2 (4): 7.

Magee A. (1996) 'BUPA accused of discriminating against elderly', *The Times*, 21 Dec.

Martin, C. E. (1990) 'A response from an educational perspective', *Nursing Clinics of North America* 25 (3): 561–8.

Mauksch, H. (1972) 'Nursing churning for change?', pp. 206–30 in H. Freeman et al. (eds), *Handbook of Medical Sociology*, 2nd edn. Englewood Cliffs NJ: Prentice Hall.

McAuliffe, E., and L. Joyce (1998) (eds) *A Healthier Future? Managed Health Care in Ireland*. Dublin: IPA.

McCarthy, G. (1997) 'Nursing and the health services', pp. 174–88 in J. Robins (ed.), *Reflections on Health Commemorating Fifty Years of the Department of Health 1947–1997*. Dublin: IPA.

McCluskey, D. (1989) *Health: People's Beliefs and Practices*. Dublin: Stationery Office.

McCluskey, D. (1997) 'Conceptions of health and illness in Ireland', pp. 51–68 in A. Cleary and M. P. Treacy (eds), *The Sociology of Health and Illness in Ireland*. Dublin: University College Dublin Press.

McCluskey, D., M. O' Keeffe and S. Slattery (1995) *The Child Health Care Service*. Dublin: Institute of Community Health Nursing.

McConkey R. and C. Conliffe (1989) 'An adult life in the community', pp. 1–10 in R. McConkey and C. Conliffe (eds), *The Person with Mental Handicap*. Dublin: St Michael's House.

McEvoy, M. (1997) 'Cross-cultural view of parents as carers', *Frontline* 32: 6.

McGann, S. (1992) *The Battle of the Nurses: A Study of Eight Women who Influenced the Development of Professional Nursing, 1880–1930*. London: Scutari.

McGeachie, J. (1999) '"Normal" development in an "abnormal" place: Sir William Wilde and the Irish School of Medicine', pp. 85–101 in E. Malcolm and G. Jones (eds), *Medicine Disease and the State in Ireland 1650–1940*. Cork: Cork University Press.

McGowan, J. (1980) *Attitude Survey of Irish Nurses*. Dublin: IPA.

McKeown, J. (1979) *The Role of Medicine*. Oxford: Oxford University Press.

McKinlay, J. (1973) 'Social networks, lay consultations and help seeking behaviour', *Social Forces* 51: 275–92.

McNally F. (1997) 'Noonan urged to relinquish role as regulator of health insurance', *The Irish Times*, 4 Jan.

McSweeney, M. and J. Kevany (1982*) Infant Feeding Practice in Ireland*. Dublin: Health Education Bureau.

McSweeney, M. and J. Kevany, (1986) *National Survey of Infant Feeding Practices in Ireland*. Dublin: Health Promotion Unit, Department of Health.

McWhinney, I. (1981) *An Introduction to Family Medicine*. Oxford: Oxford University Press.

Melia, K. (1984) 'Student nurses' construction of occupational socialisation', *Sociology of Health and Illness* 6 (2): 32–151.

Melia, K. (1987) *Learning and Working: The Occupational Socialisation of Nurses.* London: Tavistock.

Mennell, Stephen (1998) *Norbert Elias: An Introduction.* Dublin: University College Dublin Press.

Merton, R. (1957) *Social Theory and Social Structure,* rev. edn. Glencoe, Illinois: Free Press.

Miles, A. (1987) *The Mentally Ill in Contemporary Society.* Oxford: Blackwell.

Minow, M. (1987) 'When difference has its home: Group homes for the mentally retarded, equal protection and legal treatment of difference', *Harvard Civil Liberties Law Review* 22.

Moore, R. and S. Harrisson (1995) 'In poor health, socio-economic status and health chances: a review of the literature', *The Internal Journal of Research and Practice* 1 (4): 231–5.

Morgan, M., M. Calnan and N. Manning (1985) *Sociological Approaches to Health and Medicine.* London: Routledge.

Morris, J. (1993) 'Feminism and disability', *Feminist Review,* 43: 57–70.

Morse, J. (1991) 'Strategies for sampling', pp. 127–45 in J. Morse (ed.), *Qualitative Nursing Research.* London: Sage.

Mulcahy, M. and A. Reynolds (1984) *Census of Mental Handicap in the Republic of Ireland.* Dublin: Medico-Social Research Board.

Murphy, M. (1997) *Review of Indicative Drug Target Saving Scheme.* Dublin: Department of Health.

Murray, L. and P. Cooper (1988) *The Effects of Postnatal Depression on the Child.* Cambridge: Cambridge University Press.

NAMHI (National Association for People with Intellectual Disabilities) (2003) *Who Decides and How? People with Intellectual Disabilities, Legal Capacity and Decision Making.* Dublin: NAMHI.

NDA (2003) *Equal Citizens: Proposals for Disability Legislation.* Dublin: NDA www.nda.ie

NDA (2001) *Public Attitudes Towards People with Disabilities in The Republic of Ireland, Summary report on the preliminary findings of the NDA/RES survey.* www.nda.ie

NDA and Indecon (2004) *Disability and the Cost of Living.* Dublin: NDA www.nda.ie

NESC (1987) *Community Care Services: An Overview.* Dublin: NESC

NESF (1995) *Quality Delivery of Social Services.* Forum Report No. 6, Dublin: NESF.

NESF (2002) *Equity of Access to Hospital Care.* Dublin: NESF

NRB (1993) *Costs of Disability Study.* Dublin: NRB.

NRB (1998) *Costs of Disability, Study 2: Poverty among People with Disabilities.* Dublin: NRB.

National Task Force on Medical Staffing (2003) *Report* (Hanly Report). Dublin: Department of Health and Children.

Nettleton, S. (1995) *The Sociology of Health and Illness.* Cambridge: Polity.

Nolan, B. (1990) 'Socio-economic mortality differentials in Ireland', *Economic and Social Review* 21: 193–208.

Nolan, B. (1991) *The Utilisation and Financing of Health Services in Ireland.* Dublin: ESRI.

Nolan, B. (1994) 'Poverty and health inequalities', pp. 164–77 in B. Nolan and J. Callan (eds), *Poverty and Policy in Ireland.* Dublin: Gill & Macmillan.

Nolan, B. and M. Wiley (2000) *Private Practice in Irish Public Hospitals.* Dublin: Oak Tree.

Nolan M. (1997) 'Noonan gives BUPA health warning', *Evening Standard,* 9 Jan.

Norman, P. and P. Bennett (1996) 'Health locus of control', in M. Connor and P. Norman (eds), *Predicting Health Behaviour.* Buckingham: Open University Press.

Nozick, R. (1974) *Anarchy, State and Utopia.* Oxford: Oxford University Press.

Oakley, A. (1993) *Essays on Women, Medicine and Health.* Edinburgh: Edinburgh University Press.

O'Brien, E. (1984) 'The Georgian Era, 1714–1835', pp. 75–114 in E. O'Brien, A. Crookshank and G. Wolstenholme (eds), *A Portrait of Irish Medicine: An Illustrated History of Medicine in Ireland.* Dublin: Ward River Press.

O'Carroll, A. and M. O'Riordan (1996) *Counselling in General Practice: A Guide for General Practitioners.* Dublin: Irish College of General Practitioners.

O'Carroll, P. (1998) 'Blood', pp. 107–16 in M. Peillon and E. Slater (eds), *Encounters With Modern Ireland.* Dublin: IPA.

O'Connor, J., and H. Ruddle (1988) *Caring for the Elderly, Part II. The Caring Process: A Study of Carers in the Home.* Dublin: National Council for the Aged.

O'Connor P. (1998) *Emerging Voices: Women in Contemporary Irish Society.* Dublin: IPA.

O'Connor, S. (1987) *Report on Community Care.* Dublin: NESC

O'Donoghue-Woods, M. (1993) 'Costing the halo: The effects of compulsory altruism on the lives of mothers with severely handicapped adult children.' MA thesis, University College Dublin.

O'Donovan, O., and D. Casey (1995) 'Converting patients into consumers: consumerism and the charter of rights for hospital patients', *Irish Journal of Sociology* 5: 43–66.

Ogden, I. (1996) *Health Psychology.* Buckingham: Open University Press.

O'Kelly, K. (1989) *Thought for the Day.* Dublin: RTÉ.

Oliver, M. (1989) 'Disability and dependency: A creation of industrial societies', pp. 6–22 in L. Barton, (ed.), *Disability and Dependency.* London: Falmer Press.

Oliver, M. (1991) 'Speaking out: disabled people and state welfare', pp. 156–62 in G. Dalley, (ed.), *Disability and Social Policy.* London: Policy Studies Institute.

Oliver, Michael (1990) *The Politics of Disablement.* London: Macmillan.

O'Mahony, P. (2002) 'Intellectual disability and the criminal justice system', *Frontline* 50: 18–19.

Ó Moráin, P. (2000a) 'People turn to St Vincent de Paul to help pay doctors', *The Irish Times*, 24 November.

Ó Moráin, P. (2000b) 'Simple questions reveal truth of public healthcare', *The Irish Times*, 24 November.

Ormian, M. and R. Ormian (1998) 'Home from home', *Rett News* (Spring).

O'Sullivan, F. (1964) 'An exciting age', *Irish Nurse* 1: 8–12.

O'Sullivan, K. (1999) 'Irish infants are being given solids too early', *The Irish Times*, 31 August.

Painter, A. (1995) 'Health visitor identification of postnatal depression', *Health Visitor* 68 (4): 138–40.

Palmer, G. (1988) *The Politics of Breastfeeding*. London: Pandora.

Parsons, Talcott (1951) *The Social System*. Glencoe Ill.: Free Press.

Payer, L. (1988) *Medicine and Culture: Varieties of Treatment in the United States, England, West Germany and France*. New York: Penguin.

Pendleton, D., T. Schofield, P. Tate and P. Havelock (1984) *The Consultation: An Approach to Learning and Teaching*. Oxford: Oxford University Press.

Popay, J., G. Williams, C. Thomas and A. Gatrell (1998) 'Theorising inequalities in health: the place of lay knowledge', *Sociology of Health and Illness* 20: 619–44.

Porter, S. (1997) 'Why should nurses bother with sociology?', pp. 15–29 in A. Cleary and M. P. Treacy (eds), *The Sociology of Health and Illness in Ireland*. Dublin: University College Dublin Press.

Prins, A. (1990) 'Community-based services the key to integration and participation', *Frontline* Summer.

Rajan, L. (1993) 'The contribution of professional support, information and consistent correct advice to successful breast feeding', *Midwifery* 9.

Rawls, J. (1972) *A Theory of Justice*. Cambridge MA: Harvard University Press.

Reeder, L.G. (1972) 'The patient-client as a consumer: Some observations on the changing professional-client relationship', *Journal of Health and Social Behaviour*, Dec: 407.

Rees, P. (1995) 'Beating the baby blues', *The Irish Times*, 9 May.

Rees Jones, Ian (1999) *Professional Power and the Need for Health Care*. (Aldershot: Ashgate).

Rees Jones, Ian (2003) 'Health promotion and the new public health', pp. 265–76 in G. Scambler (ed.), *Sociology as Applied to Medicine*. London: W.B. Saunders.

Review Group on Health and Personal Social Services for People with Physical and Sensory Disabilities (1996) *Towards an Independent Future*. Dublin: Stationery Office.

Reynolds, J. (1992) *Grangegorman, Psychiatric Care in Dublin since 1815*. Dublin: IPA.

Rice, T. (1998) *The Economics of Health Reconsidered*. Chicago: Health Administration Press.

Ritzer, G. (1996) *Sociological Theory*. New York: McGraw-Hill.

Robins, J. (1986) *Fools and Mad: A History of the Insane in Ireland*. Dublin: IPA.

Robins, J. (1995) *The Miasma: Epidemic and Panic in Nineteenth Century Ireland.* Dublin: IPA.

Robins, J. (1997) (ed.) *Reflections on Health.* Dublin: Department of Health.

Robins, J. (2000) 'The Irish nurse in the early 1900s', pp. 11–27 in J. Robins (ed.), *Nursing and Midwifery in Ireland in the Twentieth Century.* Dublin: An Bórd Altranais.

Robinson, D. (1978) *Patients, Practitioners, and Medical Care: Aspects of Medical Sociology.* London: Heinemann.

Robinson S., T. Murrells, G. Hickey, M. Clinton and A. Tingle (2003) *A Tale of Two Courses: Comparing Careers and Competencies of Nurses Prepared via Three-Year Degree and Three-Year Diploma Courses.* London: King's College London Nursing Research Unit http://www.kcl.ac.uk/nursing/nru/nru_res_rep.html.

Rogers, E. (1995) *The Diffusion of Innovations,* 4th edn. New York: Free Press.

Rosenstock, I. (1966) 'Why people use health services', *Milbank Memorial Fund Quarterly* 44: 94–127.

Salvage, J. (1990) 'The theory and practice of new nursing', *Nursing Times* 84 (4): 42–5.

Scambler, A. (2003) 'Women and health', pp. 124–45 in G. Scambler (ed.), *Sociology as Applied to Medicine,* 5th edn. London: Saunders.

Scambler, A., G. Scambler and D. Craig (1981) 'Kinship and friendship networks and women's demand for primary care', *Journal of Royal College of General Practitioners* 26: 746–50.

Scambler, G. (1997) 'Health and illness behaviour', pp. 35–46 in G. Scambler (ed.), *Sociology As Applied To Medicine,* 4th edn. London: Saunders.

Scambler, G. (2003) *Sociology as Applied to Medicine,* 5th edn. London: W. B. Saunders.

Scambler, G. and A. Scambler (1995) 'Social change and health promotion among sex workers in London', *Health Promotion International* 10: 17–24.

Seekamp, G. (1996) 'BUPA v VHI: How do they compare?', *Sunday Business Post,* 24 Nov.

Seekamp G. (1997) 'BUPA launched products without government check', *Sunday Business Post,* 5 Jan.

Seekamp G. and T. Harding (1997) 'Chaos rules in "new era"', *Sunday Business Post,* 5 Jan.

Seeman, M. and J. Seeman (1983) 'Health behaviour and personal autonomy: a longitudinal study of the sense of control in illness', *Journal of Health and Social Behaviour* 24: 144–60.

Sellers, E. T. (2000) 'Images of a new sub-culture in the Australian university: perceptions of non-nurse academics of the discipline of nursing', *Higher Education* 43: 157–72.

Shannon, W. (1983) *Profile of an Irish General Practice: An Analysis of Morbidity and a Selective Clinical Audit.* Cork: University College Cork.

Sheeran, P. and C. Abraham (1996) 'The health belief model', pp. 23–61 in M. Connor and P. Norman (eds), *Predicting Health Behaviour.* Buckingham: Open University Press.

Shilling, Chris (1993) *The Body and Social Theory.* London: Sage.

Simons, H., J. B. Clarke, M. Gobbi and G. Long (1998) *Nurse Education and Training Evaluation in Ireland.* Dublin: Department of Health.

Starr, Paul (1982) *The Social Transformation of American Medicine.* New York: Basic Books.

Stewart, D. and P. Shamdasani (1990) *Focus Groups: Theory and Practice.* London: Sage.

St Michael's House (2002) *Five-Year Plan, 2002–2006.* Dublin: St Michael's House.

Stone, D. (1984) *The Disabled State.* London: Macmillan.

Strong, P. (1977) 'Medical errands: a discussion of routine patient work', pp. 38–54 in A. Davis and G. Horobin (eds), *Medical Encounters.* London: Croom Helm.

Sunday Tribune (1997) 'BUPA expected to target profitable', 5 Jan.

Sussman.G. (1982) *Selling Mother's Milk: The Wet-Nursing Business in France, 1715–1914.* Urbana: University of Illinois Press.

Sweetman, R. (1979) *On Our Backs: Sexual Attitudes in a Changing Ireland.* London: Pan.

Szasz, T. and M. H. Hollender (1956) 'A contribution to the philosophy of medicine: the basis models of the doctor–patient relationship', *American Medical Association, Archives of Internal Medicine* 97: 586.

Tormey, B. (2003) *A Cure for the Crisis: Irish Healthcare in Context.* Dublin: Blackwater Press.

Townsend, P. and N. Davidson (1982) *Inequalities in Health: The Black Report.* Harmondsworth: Penguin.

Townsend, P. and N. Davidson (1992) 'The Black Report', pp. 29–213 in P. Townsend, N. Davidson and M. Whitehead (eds), *Inequalities in Health.* London: Penguin.

Treacy, M. (1987) 'In the pipeline: A qualitative study of general nurse training with special reference to nurses' role in health education', PhD thesis, University of London.

Tubridy, I. (1995) *Views from the Inside,* prepared for the Commission on the Status of People with Disabilities.

Tuckett, D. (1976) 'Introduction', pp. 1–40 in D. Tuckett (ed.), *An Introduction to Medical Sociology.* London: Tavistock.

Tudor Hart, J. (1971) 'The inverse care law', *The Lancet,* 1: 405–12.

Tussing, A. D. (1985) *Irish Medical Care Resources: An Economic Analysis.* Dublin: ESRI.

Van de Ven W. P. M. M. (1991) 'Perestrojka in the Dutch health care system', *European Economic Review* 35: 430–40.

Van de Ven W. P. M. M. and R. C. J. A. van Vliet (1992) 'How can we prevent cream skimming in a competitive health insurance market?', pp. 23–46 in P. Zwiefel and H.E. Frech III (eds), *Health Economics Worldwide.* Amsterdam: Kluwer.

VHI (1996) *A Guide to Plans ABCDE.* Dublin: VHI.

Wadsworth, M., W. Butterfield and R. Blaney (1971) *Health and Sickness: The Choice of Treatment.* London: Tavistock.

Wall, V. and D. Murphy (1996) 'Noonan asks BUPA to justify plans under community rating', *Irish Independent*, 21 Dec.

Wallston, B., K. Wallston, G. Kaplan and S. Maides (1976) 'Development and validation of Health Locus of Control (HLC) scale', *Journal of Consulting and Clinical Psychology* 44: 580–85.

Wallston, K. and B. Wallston (1978) 'Development of multidimensional Health Locus of Control (MHLC) Scales', *Health Education Monographs* 6: 160.

Walzer, Michael (1983) *Spheres of Justice: A Defense of Pluralism and Equality*. New York: Basic Books.

Watson Wyatt Worldwide (2003) *Audit of Structures and Functions in the Health System* (Prospectus Report). Dublin: Stationery Office.

Webb, A. (1968) *The Clean Sweep*. London: George G. Harrap.

Webb, C. (1992) 'What is nursing?', *British Journal of Nursing* 1 (11): 567–8.

Weber, Max. (1968) (1921) *Economy and Society*. New York: Bedminster.

Weiss, G. L. and L. E. Lonnquist (1999) *The Sociology of Health, Healing and Illness*, 3rd edn. Englewood Cliffs NJ: Prentice-Hall.

Whelan, C. T. (ed.) (1994) *Values and Social Change in Ireland*. Dublin: Gill & Macmillan.

Whitehead, M. (1988) *The Health Divide*. London: Health Education Council.

Whitehead, M. (1992) 'The Health Divide' in P. Townsend, N. Davidson and M. Whitehead (eds), *Inequalities in Health*. London: Penguin.

Whyte, J. (1980) *Church and State in Modern Ireland, 1923–1979*, 2nd edn. Dublin: Gill & Macmillan.

Wilcock, F. (1995) 'Sugars and spice', *Health Visitor* 68 (5): 181–2.

Wiley, M. (1997) 'Irish health policy in perspective', pp. 213–27 in F. Ó Muircheartaigh (ed.), *Ireland In The Coming Times*. Dublin: IPA.

Wiley, M. (1998) 'Health expenditure trends in Ireland: past, present and future', pp. 69–82 in A. Leahy and M. Wiley (eds), *The Irish Health System in the 21st Century*. Dublin: Oak Tree.

Wiley, M. (2002) 'Huge cash injections into health service cannot continue indefinitely', *The Irish Times*, 17 Apr. 2002.

Wiley, M. and B. Merriman (1996) *Women and Health Care in Ireland*. Dublin: ESRI.

Witz, A. (1992) *Professions and Patriarchy*. London: Routledge.

Wolf, J. (1996) 'Withholding their due: the dispute between Ireland and Great Britain over unemployed insurance payments to conditionally landed Irish wartime volunteer workers', *Saothar* 21: 39–45.

Wolfensberger, W. (1972) *The Principle of Normalisation in Human Services*. Toronto: National Institute on Mental Retardation.

Woods, G. (1978) 'Primary health care', pp. 66–89 in P. Brearley, J. Gibbons, A. Miles, Topliss and G. Woods (eds), *The Social Context of Health Care*. Oxford: Blackwell & Mott.

Woods, M. (1997) *Costing the Halo*. NRB Occasional Paper. Dublin: NRB.

Working Group on Health (1996) *Working Paper on Health*, prepared for the Commission on the Status of People with Disabilities.

Working Party on Prescribing and Dispensing in the General Medical Service (1974) *Report*. Dublin: Stationery Office.

Working Party on the General Medical Service (1984) *Report*. Dublin: Stationery Office.

World Health Organisation (1986) 'Life-styles and health', *Social Science and Medicine* 22: 117–24.

World Health Organisation (1989) *Protecting, Promoting and Supporting Breast-feeding: The Special Role of the Maternity Services*. Geneva: WHO.

World Health Organisation (n.d.) *Definition of Disability*.

Wouters, Cas (1977) 'Informalisation and the civilising process', pp. 437–53 in P. Gleichmann et al. (eds), *Human Figurations: Essays for Norbert Elias*. Amsterdam: Stichting Amsterdams Sociologisch Tijdschrift.

Wouters, Cas (1986) 'Formalisation and informalisation: changing tension balances in civilising processes', *Theory, Culture and Society* 3 (2): 1–18.

Wren, M.-A. (2003) *Unhealthy State*. Dublin: New Island.

Zelizer, V. A. R. (1985) *Pricing the Priceless Child: the Changing Social Value of Children*. New York: Basic Books.

Zelizer, V. A. R. (1994) *The Social Meaning of Money*. New York: Basic Books.

Zola, I. K. (1966) 'Culture and symptoms – an analysis of patients' presenting complaints', *American Sociological Review* 31: 615–30.

Zola, I. K. (1972) 'Medicine as an institution of social control', *Sociological Review* 20: 487–504.

Zola, I. K. (1978) 'Medicine as an institution of social control: the medicalising of society', pp. 254–60 in D. Tuckett and J. M. Kaufert (eds), *Basic Readings in Medical Sociology*. London: Tavistock.

Index